NATURAL PROGESTERONE

NATURAL PROGESTERONE

The natural way to alleviate
symptoms of menopause, PMS, and
other hormone-related problems

AnnA Rushton and Dr Shirley A Bond

Thorsons
An Imprint of HarperCollins*Publishers*

Thorsons
An Imprint of HarperCollins*Publishers*
77–85 Fulham Palace Road,
Hammersmith, London W6 8JB

Published by Thorsons 1999
5 7 9 10 8 6 4

A catalogue record for this book
is available from the British Library

ISBN 0 7225 3766 2

Printed in Great Britain by
Creative Print and Design (Wales), Ebbw Vale

Contents

Foreword

Writing the Foreword to this book, *Natural Progesterone*, is a twofold pleasure. First, it is a pleasure to contribute to a book that grew, as it were, literally from the authors' hands-on experience of using natural progesterone to restore hormone balance in their health counselling of women. Given the importance of progesterone and the continuing obduracy of conventional medicine in this regard, we need more books to reach more women to create the demand that will restore progesterone to its rightful place in hormone balancing. It is a sad fact that natural (i.e. bio-identical) progesterone has been neglected and ignored for more than 40 years in favour of the less effective, more toxic synthetic substitutes (progestogens). As a result, women must educate themselves on this matter and thereby become their own best health advocate in matters of hormone balancing. Thus the need for this book.

Secondly, I find pleasure in the fact that the authors are so well qualified. AnnA Rushton and Dr Shirley Bond both early on instantly grasped the significance of progesterone deficiency and its corollary, oestrogen dominance, in the health of women. AnnA Rushton brings to her peer counselling a sound understanding of hormone balance combined with wide experience in health writing and a commonsense approach to stress management, all administered with gusto and practicality. I know Dr Shirley Bond to be a remarkably intelligent, caring and insightful physician whose ministration to patients is a delightful blend of solid scientific reasoning and good cheer. Her leadership and broad experience in using natural progesterone in women is perhaps unrivalled in the UK. Their combined experience, the success they have witnessed, and their personal attributes make them the ideal authors for this practical and insightful guide to the role of natural progesterone in women's health.

Progesterone deficiency is a bit different from other important illnesses. It lacks, for instance, any obvious signs such as the rash of measles or chickenpox, or fever or pallor, or specific aches and pains. But it and its corollary, oestrogen dominance, are just as important, if not more, than most other illnesses. It can result, for example, in breast, ovary or endometrial cancer, fibrocystic breasts, weight gain, infertility, early miscarriage, osteoporosis, autoimmune disorders, water retention, loss of libido and more rapid ageing. The clinical diagnosis of progesterone deficiency may be too subtle for catastrophe-oriented physicians, but it is not less sure, thanks to modern laboratory tests. It is the women who will first recognize progesterone deficiency and oestrogen dominance – they know their own bodies. It is the women who, on sensing a hormone change, will have to remind their doctors to check their luteal phase progesterone levels in addition to the usual estradiol, FSH or thyroid tests. The patient will teach her doctor to obtain saliva hormone assays, rather than serum (or plasma) tests, to monitor the progesterone absorption from transdermal creams, since such testing is not yet standard in the lexicon of conventional medicine.

The results of the proper use of progesterone are likewise subtle but profound: the breast cancer is prevented, sleep patterns return to normal, PMS gradually fades, energy levels rise, thinking becomes less rattled, the bone will not fracture, or the libido returns and the marriage is saved. The doctor may not appreciate the importance of these subtle changes, but the woman does. Hundreds of them write to me, and I'm sure also to Dr Bond and AnnA Rushton, saying 'Thank you for giving me back my life.'

Thus the need for this book.

John R Lee, MD
Sebastopol, California
October 1998

Introduction

Feeling healthy, vital, full of energy. This is how most of us would like to live. Much of the time we are 'mostly all right', sometimes we are fairly ill, and too often many women face life-threatening illnesses such as cancer at an earlier age than we had ever thought possible. It is too easy to dismiss this as 'what happens'; our health is too important for us not to pay attention to what will make us whole, balanced and free from hormonal problems.

There are many areas we can look at in relation to our health; we know we ought to exercise, eat properly and try to live a balanced life. For many of us, though, that balance does not extend to our hormonal health. Women's internal balance is seriously compromised by the way we live, the drug regimes such as the Pill and HRT that we have become accustomed to being prescribed, and environmental factors over which we have no control.

We do, however, have control over our own bodies. So many of the problems that beset women throughout their lives, from PMS to hysterectomy, breast cancer to osteoporosis, can all be directly attributed to the imbalance in our bodies between the hormones oestrogen and progesterone.

There has been much debate about the role of oestrogen, and many claims made as to its beneficial effect on women's health, particularly at menopause. Much less has been heard about the vital necessity of oestrogen being properly balanced by sufficient progesterone. Most of that debate has been ignored by many doctors who have remained determinedly unaware of the crucial role progesterone has for women's health. It is their women patients who have taken the responsibility for finding a solution to their hormonal health problems. Over the last few years women have been finding and passing on simple and straightforward information which can help them, and other women, to better health.

I have been writing about all aspects of alternative health care since 1988, and after meeting John Lee MD – the first doctor to really make women aware of the need for progesterone – I became instrumental in providing information on this vital topic to as many women as possible. It was for this reason I founded Woman to Woman – in order to help women pass on this information to each other. For several years now, Dr Shirley Bond and I have been giving talks to women about their health, and it has been heartening and inspiring to see the dedication with which some of these women have battled on to find a cure, or a reason for, their hormonal illnesses. Progesterone is not a 'magic bullet' which will cure all women's problems, but it is a totally essential hormone for women's health and its role has been sadly under-emphasized and undervalued by the medical profession.

The topics we cover in this book are those raised at our seminars. There are several excellent books on hormone balance, but none so far that has attempted to answer the questions that women have been asking their own doctors and each other in a concerted effort to give themselves the best of health. We would like to thank all the women who have asked us questions, especially the ones we didn't have an answer for, as it has allowed us to check out the worldwide research on progesterone and investigate the misinformation that is so common. We have not answered all the questions about what progesterone can do – I suspect we are at the beginning of actually starting to find that out – but our purpose is to share the information we have with as many women, and their doctors, as possible.

Thank you for helping us to do that.

AnnA Rushton
November 1998

CHAPTER 1

A Woman's Hormone History

Our hormone story starts in the womb, long before we are born. When a female embryo is only about 21 days old, and measures a mere 2 millimetres in length, her hormonal life starts. At this stage the embryo does not have any organs that can be specifically recognized, but a heartbeat can be seen under a microscope.

Cells from what is known as the yolk sac of the embryo migrate into an area of the embryo where the ovaries will eventually develop. These cells divide, and by about the fifth month of the pregnancy a female foetus will have ovaries containing around seven million eggs, or ova. Incredibly, from the time all our eggs have been produced, even before the foetus has reached maturity, these eggs begin to die. At the time of a girl's birth, each ovary is left with only about two million eggs, and by puberty the number will have reduced even more to between five hundred thousand and two hundred thousand. Of these, only a fraction will eventually ovulate. We do not know what the explanation is for this seemingly wasteful process.

THE MONTHLY CYCLE

The ovaries remain inactive until puberty. For most girls this usually occurs during the teens, but may be earlier or later. It is not known what triggers puberty, but an area of the brain known as the hypothalamus starts to secrete a hormone known as the Gonadotrophic Stimulating Hormone. This hormone affects the pituitary, which in response starts to secrete another hormone known as Follicular Stimulating Hormone (FSH). This hormone affects the ovary and, as its name suggests, stimulates the follicles of the ovary. The follicles contain immature ova and, under the effect of FSH, a number of these follicles begin to develop. Soon one of these follicles becomes more mature than the others. As it develops, the cells inside this follicle – known as granulosa cells – secrete oestrogen. The oestrogen levels rise, and when they reach a certain level, which will vary from woman to woman, the pituitary stops secreting FSH and starts to secrete another hormone known as Leuteinizing Hormone (LH). Within a day or two of this change the follicle bursts and the egg is expelled. This is the process of ovulation, which should occur normally each month.

At this point, the granulosa cells of the follicle stop making so much oestrogen, and start making progesterone. The area from which the egg was expelled is known as the corpus luteum, or yellow body, because it does indeed turn yellow in colour. The other developing follicles in both ovaries stop developing and disappear. If the egg is fertilized it secretes a hormone known as Human Chorionic Gonadotrophin. This hormone ensures that the ovary continues to make large quantities of progesterone to prepare the uterus for a pregnancy. If the egg is not fertilized, no Human Chorionic Gonadotrophic hormone is secreted, the ovary stops producing progesterone and the cycle starts again.

The levels of oestrogen and progesterone produced during this cycle also have an effect on the uterus itself. During the first part of this hormonal cycle, the increasing amounts of oestrogen being produced build up the endometrium (the lining of the uterus). The progesterone also has an effect here, as it matures and makes ready the endometrium to receive the fertilized egg, which will be able to implant and form a placenta, which also in its turn will then produce progesterone.

The role of progesterone is vital. It ensures that the lining of the uterus is mature and that it is not shed, thus enabling a young embryo to survive. It is this role of promoting pregnancy that gives this hormone its name – 'pro' meaning in favour of, and 'gestation' meaning pregnancy. If fertilization of an egg does not occur and the secretion of progesterone by the corpus luteum stops, then the lining of the uterus is shed and a woman experiences her normal monthly period or bleed.

THE END OF THE HORMONE CYCLE

When menopause is reached, the cycle stops. There is no more ovulation or monthly bleed. As with puberty, it is not known what causes the change in the hormone pattern. If you remember that our ovaries are actually older than we are, it may be that an ageing ovary simply stops responding to the pituitary hormones. It may be that some built-in mechanism in the brain affects the pituitary via the hypothalamus, so that the FSH and LH no longer have the same effect. In any case, as it is essential that a mother survives long enough to rear her young to maturity, the fact that the way in which the human female ceases being reproductive long before she is too old to cope with childbearing has ensured the survival of the human species.

Nature's plan seems to be for this cycle to continue from puberty to menopause without ceasing, except for pregnancies, and without problems. Sadly, this does not seem to be what happens to women today.

WHAT CAN ALTER OUR HORMONE BALANCE

First we need to be clear about the effects that progesterone and oestrogen have in the body. We are indebted to Dr John Lee for the work he has done in identifying and publicizing the vital role of progesterone. The following is taken with his permission from a list he produced at a seminar given in London in September 1998:

The Effects of Oestrogen

creates proliferative endometrium
breast stimulation
increases body fat
aids salt and fluid retention
contributes to depression and headaches
interferes with thyroid hormone
impairs blood sugar control
increases blood clotting
decreases libido
contributes to the loss of zinc and retention of copper
reduces oxygen levels in all cells
causes endometrial cancer
increases risk of breast cancer
slightly restrains osteoclast function, in order to slow
  down bone loss
reduces vascular tone
triggers autoimmune disease

The Effects of Progesterone

maintains secretory endometrium
protects against fibrocystic breasts

helps use fat for energy
natural diuretic
natural anti-depressant
facilitates thyroid hormone action
normalizes blood sugar levels
normalizes blood clotting
increases libido
normalizes zinc and copper levels
restores proper cell oxygen levels
prevents endometrial cancer
helps prevent breast cancer
stimulates osteoblast bone-building
improves vascular tone
turns off autoimmune diseases
necessary for survival of embryo
precursor of corticosterone production.

It is clear that these two hormones are intended to balance each other and work in harmony for maximum hormone health. Sadly, when they do not it is usually the result of interference from artificial hormones, drug regimes, lifestyle and environmental pollution.

The problem of excess oestrogen has been recognized by some doctors since the 1930s, but it was not realized that the real importance lay in the ratio of oestrogen to progesterone, not just their actual levels. It was Dr John Lee, an American doctor in general practice, who first widely publicized it and gave it the name of *oestrogen dominance*. This name came into common usage from his first book published in the mid-1990s – *Natural Progesterone: Multiple Roles of a Remarkable Hormone* – which he wrote to alert other doctors to the true importance of progesterone levels for women's hormone health. In fact it has been women who have taken up the challenge of his work and used it to help them identify for themselves when they were receiving unopposed oestrogen, or an excess of oestrogen not properly balanced with sufficient progesterone.

Symptoms of Oestrogen Dominance

acceleration of the ageing process
allergies, including asthma, rashes, sinus congestion
autoimmune disorders
breast tenderness
cervical dysplasia
cold hands and feet, relating to thyroid dysfunction
decreased sex drive
depression with anxiety or agitation
dry eyes
early onset of menstruation
fat gain, especially around the abdomen, hips and thighs
fatigue
fibrocystic breasts
gallbladder disease
hair loss
headaches
hypoglycaemia
inability to focus
increase blood clotting
increased risk of strokes
infertility
irregular menstruation
irritability
insomnia
memory loss
miscarriage
mood swings
osteoporosis
pre-menopausal bone loss
PMS

sluggish metabolism
uterine cancer
uterine fibroids
water retention, bloating

POLLUTION

One of the least-recognized causes of oestrogen dominance is the environmental effect of pollution. Most people are aware that we have been polluting our environment for many years and upsetting the balance of nature. However, there are not too many who realize that a great deal of the pollution consists of substances that are – or can become – xeno-oestrogens. Xeno-oestrogens are chemicals which have the characteristic of behaving like oestrogens and attaching themselves to oestrogen receptors. The fact that they are now so widespread in the environment is because they are the breakdown products of many processes involved in the petrochemical and plastics industries. They are even exuded from plastics (for example furniture, carpets, underlay, some paints and plastic water bottles), especially if they are warmed in any way.

These xeno-oestrogens attach themselves to oestrogen receptors in the body and produce stronger effects than oestrogen itself. They are also difficult for the body to remove from the receptors, so they stay in the body and have prolonged effects. This is unlike phyto-oestrogens (oestrogens found in plants), which also attach to the body's oestrogen receptors but seem to have weaker effects than oestrogen.

The environment is further polluted by the passing of oestrogens into the water supply. These come from women who are taking the contraceptive pill and HRT. We are told that these are removed from our drinking water when it is recycled, but many experts doubt that this is completely possible.

Now we have an overview of the life history of our hormones, and what can cause problems to arise. In the following chapters we will look at the individual problems that occur at the different stages of a woman's life.

CHAPTER 2

Progesterone: What It Is and How to Use It

We can see from the preceding chapter how essential progesterone is for women's health. It may seem obvious what progesterone is, but many people – medical professionals included – will use the word progesterone when they are also describing the actions of the synthetic progestagens, or progestins as they are known in the United States. In this book, *progesterone* refers only to the natural hormone produced in the ovaries, or a supplementary form of it that is bio-identical. This means that it is recognized by the woman's own body as identical in every way to the progesterone she would produce herself. Because natural progesterone supplementation is fairly new to many, this chapter will also give guidelines on what exactly progesterone does, what forms it can be obtained in, and how we may be directed to use it.

PROGESTERONE IN THE BODY

Progesterone is a hormone which is present in both men and women. In the woman it is made in the ovary by the corpus luteum after ovulation has occurred, and also in the adrenals. In a woman the level produced daily varies, and can depend on whether she is pre-menopausal, post-menopausal or pregnant.

Average levels of progesterone produced in optimum circumstances:

Pre-menopausal woman prior to ovulation	5–10 milligrams (mg) per day
Pre-menopausal woman after ovulation	20—50 mg per day
Pregnant woman	the levels rise dramatically and can reach 400 mg per day
Post-menopausal women	10 mg per day
Men (whose progesterone is made in the adrenals and the testis)	5—15 mg per day

The levels of progesterone present on any particular day can be measured either by a blood or saliva test.

Progesterone is synthesized in the body from cholesterol via the hormone *pregnenolone*. Progesterone itself can be converted into cortico-steroids and testosterone.

Progesterone receptors are found on the cells in many tissues of the body, including those of: the uterus, cervix, vagina, brain cells, peripheral nerve myelin sheaths and bone cells. These receptors can affect many bodily functions and systems, including: temperature control, stress responses, the immune system, energy production and fat metabolism.

Progesterone also affects the behaviour of other hormones; perhaps its most vital role is in ensuring the survival of the foetus. Although it is always referred to as a sex hormone, it does not in fact impart any secondary sex characteristics.

WHY IS IT CALLED 'NATURAL' PROGESTERONE?

Natural progesterone is a name which has been acquired by the progesterone that is produced in a laboratory for putting into creams or tablets for supplementation. The word 'natural' in this context means that the progesterone made in the laboratory has exactly the same chemical structure as progesterone made in the body – meaning that it is natural to the body and fully recognized by it as identical to the progesterone produced by a woman herself. If a chemist were given a molecule of progesterone from a human body and a molecule of progesterone made in the laboratory, he or she would not be able to tell which was which from their chemical structure. The practical application of this means that when you use natural progesterone cream your body has all the enzyme systems to use the hormone properly – it will act in exactly the same way as your own progesterone would. That is to say, it will not accumulate in the body or produce side-effects.

Progesterone is made in the laboratory from *saponins*. These are steroid-like substances found in plants. The most commonly used is diosgenin, which is found in Mexican wild yams. This substance is treated in the laboratory and, in a simple three-stage cascade process, is converted into progesterone. It is then micronized, which means it is treated in such a way that the molecules do not form large structures, but remain in small groups. The advantage of this is that they can then be absorbed readily, even through the skin. This form of progesterone is fat-soluble and, as a result, is carried on the red blood cell membranes rather than in the watery blood plasma. It is released from the red cell membranes when it reaches the progesterone receptors. In order to check that you are absorbing the progesterone in a cream, you need to have saliva as well as blood tests. This is because blood levels will rise when you are using natural progesterone, and although this rise is usually taken as an indicator that a woman has sufficient progesterone, this actually indicates only that progesterone is being transported to its eventual destination. This is why a blood test is generally not an accurate assessment of true progesterone levels in the body. A saliva test, on the other hand, can measure the progesterone in its fat-soluble form, more accurately indicating whether or not absorption is taking place.

FORMS OF NATURAL PROGESTERONE AVAILABLE

Until a few years ago there was very little choice. Natural progesterone was available as a pessary, a cream or an injection. Now, with the greater interest in the vital role of this hormone for women's health, we are able to choose from a much wider range of products and new ones are currently being developed. Most of the work has been done in the US, and it is from here that the greatest range of products is still being produced.

Please note that what follows is a guide to what is available, although certain products may not be obtainable from your own doctor or in your particular country. In the UK, progesterone products are only available on prescription from a doctor, though they may be ordered directly for personal use from outside the country. Information on manufacturers and importers will be found in the Resources chapter.

TRANSDERMAL CREAMS
Transdermal creams have been shown scientifically to be readily absorbed and to produce a reliable and predictable

level of progesterone in the body. A 1.6 per cent is the form of progesterone on which most of the recently published work and research by Dr John Lee and others is based. There are many different natural progesterone creams on the market depending on which country you live in, but they fall into roughly four categories:

1 Creams which contain only progesterone in a base carrier such as vitamin E or aloe vera.
2 Creams with progesterone plus other inactive substances such as essential oils or herbs. These additions are thought to aid the absorption of the progesterone and improve the quality of the cream itself.
3 Creams which contain progesterone and various phyto-oestrogens.
4 Creams which contains progesterone and tri-oestrogen.

There are advantages and disadvantages to the combined creams. The advantages are that often the phyto-oestrogens or tri-oestrogens are also needed to control the symptoms from which you may suffer. The disadvantage is that you are unable to adjust the individual doses of either the oestrogens or the progesterone. If you increase or decrease the amount of cream you use then you are affecting both hormones, and it could be that while the ratio of the doses contained in the cream is suitable for many people, it may not be correct for you.

The percentage of progesterone in the creams can also vary, and range from a 1.6 per cent cream which contains approximately 850 milligrams (mg) progesterone in a 2-oz tube or jar, up to a 10 per cent cream. This is obviously a huge difference; you need to check the amount you are being given. The amount of progesterone in the combined creams also varies from manufacturer to manufacturer. It is important that you know how many milligrams of progesterone there is in each ounce of cream, rather than the percentage of progesterone it contains. The reason for this is that there is sometimes confusion as to whether the percentage is calculated on a weight or volume basis.

There are no reported side-effects with the creams. The only drawback can be that they are not suitable in the few cases which require very high doses of natural progesterone supplementation – for instance in PMS.

At the time of writing, no progesterone cream has been licensed for use in the UK, but it is believed one will be available during 1999.

SUBLINGUAL OIL
Progesterone is also available in the form of an oil. This is usually taken by putting drops of it under the tongue. It is a useful way to take progesterone when a rapid response is required. The drawback is that, because it acts quickly in the body, it is also removed from the bloodstream just as fast and so is not really suitable for maintenance and long-term oestrogen balance.

SUBLINGUAL TABLETS OR LOZENGES
Progesterone in this form comes in a wide range of dosages. It is readily absorbed from under the tongue, so low doses are effective because the progesterone is absorbed directly into the bloodstream and does not have to pass through the liver before it reaches its target organs.

TABLETS AND CAPSULES
This form of progesterone is taken by mouth and is absorbed via the digestive tract. As a result, higher doses are needed to produce the same effect produced by transdermal or sublingual routes, because the progesterone has to pass through the liver where some will be broken down before it reaches the target organs.

This is often the most effective form when high doses are needed. The amount of progesterone which can be administered this way varies from 25 mg up to 400 mg or more.

At present there are no licensed progesterone tablets or capsules in the UK, but at the time of writing there is one being put up for approval by the FDA (Food and Drug Administration) in the USA.

SUPPOSITORIES

Suppositories for rectal or vaginal use have been licensed and prescribed for many years. They are available in the UK as Cyclogest and their progesterone content is either 200 or 400 mg. They are often prescribed by doctors for PMS, and after the implantation of an embryo in some IVF programmes.

The problem with this form of progesterone can be the rather high dose, which can lead to side-effects.

VAGINAL GEL

A 4 per cent progesterone vaginal gel is also licenced and available on prescription. It is manufactured under the brand name Crinone. It can be used to balance oestrogen for women on traditional HRT. The problem here, as with the Cyclogest, can be the high dosage. The method of application and delivery is also not as easy to regulate as the creams.

INJECTION

There is a form of progesterone available for injection. The main problem with its use is that the absorption from the injection site seems to be unpredictable.

Dosages and Regimes

There is often a great deal of confusion as to the dose of natural progesterone that should be given, how it should be used, and when it should be used.

The first thing to remember is that in a normal menstrual cycle progesterone is present in very small quantities during the first half of the cycle, rises rapidly to high levels immediately after ovulation and remains high for 14 days. If fertilization of the egg has not occurred, then the level of progesterone drops suddenly on or about day 14 and menstruation results. If, however, fertilization of the egg has occurred and a pregnancy results, then the levels of progesterone remain high. Oestrogen levels tend to remain high throughout the cycle.

HORMONE TESTING

If you want to know what your hormones are doing you can find out by having a blood or saliva test done. The best time of the cycle to do a single blood test is around seven to ten days before your period commences. This should show a high progesterone level to confirm ovulation. If you suspect that your progesterone levels fall off earlier in the cycle than they should, then you can repeat the test five or six days later.

Saliva tests can also be done to indicate your hormone levels, and this is the method suggested by Dr John Lee as being the most accurate monitor of progesterone levels. Again, if you are doing a one-off test then the days suggested for the blood tests apply. It is, however, easier with the salivary tests to do a series of tests throughout the month and see more accurately what is happening throughout the cycle.

At the time of writing these tests are carried out in the US at Aeron Life Cycles; samples are sent to them from all over the world. You do not need a doctor's referral in order to request these tests (details in the Resources chapter). This laboratory also returns your results with advice as to when you need to supplement with natural progesterone.

A sensible question to ask, though, is whether you need to have your levels tested at all. It is very important to remember that all hormone tests are limited in that they can only really tell what your hormone levels are on the day that you take them. It is quite possible to do the tests one month and receive a result that says you are definitely menopausal, and to repeat them the next month and have normal levels which show you are still ovulating. This is why it is essential to interpret these results in the light of your symptoms and not just go on the hormone levels themselves. For many women, checking the list of oestrogen dominance symptoms is as accurate —and considerably cheaper – than undergoing a series of tests. Blood tests are available through your doctor (and therefore free in the UK), but saliva tests are something you would normally have to pay for yourself.

Dosage

For the majority of women, it is the transdermal creams that are most helpful for hormonal symptoms as they are given in the physiological dose that mimics that which would be produced by the woman's own ovaries. Most creams come with dosage instructions, but the following is a guide for women taking a standard progesterone cream (a 1.6 per cent cream which contains approximately 850 mg progesterone in a 2-oz tube or jar, such as Pro-Gest). For controlling symptoms of oestrogen dominance it is sensible to start supplementing initially with a progesterone cream that does not contain additional ingredients, as this may confuse the picture as to how progesterone is controlling your symptoms. For creams containing other ingredients or of a higher concentration of progesterone than 1.6 per cent, the dosage would need to be adjusted, so please follow the instructions provided with the cream and discuss it with your prescribing physician.

The following dosage regimes are a suggested guide only:

WOMEN WHO ARE STILL HAVING PERIODS

It is usually best to confine the supplementation of natural progesterone to the second half of the cycle. If you do this you are less likely to interfere with ovulation. The dosage normally used is 15–20 mg twice a day. Progesterone creams are usually supplied with a prescribing leaflet which gives general indications as to how much to use to obtain this dosage.

WOMEN WHO HAVE STOPPED HAVING PERIODS

At this time, women are usually supplementing with natural progesterone to treat oestrogen-dominance symptoms. These are best treated by supplementing with natural progesterone daily, except for five or six days each calender month. Many women simply choose the first week of a month as their 'natural progesterone-free' days, as this is the easiest to remember. This few days' break without progesterone each month is to allow the uterus to bleed if any lining has built up, and to prevent the receptors becoming unresponsive to the progesterone.

The dosage for this group should be approximately 15 mg twice a day.

WOMEN WHO ARE HAVING IRREGULAR PERIODS

When this is the situation it is often difficult to work out a regime. The principle to follow is that you are aiming to use the cream for three weeks out of every four. The week when you do not use the cream should be the week when you have, or would expect to have, your period. Confusion arises when you have followed this regime and used the cream for three weeks, but when you then stop for a week you do not have a period. Then, a few days after you restart the cream, your period appears. What should you do? You should stop the cream again for five days, and then restart again for three weeks. If bleeding keeps occurring, so that you seem unable to use the cream for more than a few days, you should try one of these two regimes:

1 You should stop the cream for three or four weeks, then start again, or

2 Continue using the cream for three weeks then have one week off, regardless of your bleeding pattern. When the bleeding settles down, you then try to fit your use of cream to the pattern of your bleeding.

Whichever regime you and your practitioner decide on, the dosage should be 15–20 mg twice a day unless the bleeding is difficult to control. If this is the case then you may need to use a higher dosage for a while. If irregular bleeding continues, or starts after your periods have stopped for a while, you should always seek medical advice to establish that you do not have a serious problem other than a hormone imbalance which is causing the bleeding.

It is always best if you can obtain the help of a practitioner if you have difficulty working out your regime or dosage.

Progesterone Uses and Types: Questions and Answers

ON THE INSTRUCTIONS WITH MY CREAM IT SAYS I SHOULD ROTATE THE SITES I USE IT. I AM NOT QUITE SURE WHAT THIS MEANS?
Simply that you do not want to put the cream onto the same place every day. Most women who are using the cream experiment to find their own routine, but a simple way is to think of using it where the skin is thinnest and it will be most easily absorbed.

Each day you want to put the cream in a different place. You could start on day one with the face, then on other days use the neck, upper chest, palms of the hands, lower arms, upper arms, stomach or inner thighs. That will give you more than seven different places to put the cream, and as there are seven days in the week, it should work out. Also, splitting the dose so you are having half in the morning and half in the evening usually helps absorption, unless you are specifically directed otherwise.

I RUB THE CREAM ON, BUT IT DOESN'T SEEM TO SINK IN PROPERLY. AM I DOING SOMETHING WRONG?

The answer is not to rub so hard. It isn't necessary. Just gently stroke it on with the tips of your fingers. If you rub hard it seems that the cream may 'lather up' and it can be more difficult then to get it absorbed.

IS THERE ANY DIFFERENCE BETWEEN USING NATURAL PROGESTERONE AS A CREAM OR AS A PESSARY OR VAGINAL GEL?

The transdermal creams, the pessaries and the vaginal gels all contain progesterone. The progesterone in them all is identical to progesterone produced in the body. There is a considerable difference, however, in the amount of progesterone in the creams and in the pessaries or gel. The creams may be of different strengths but the dosage is usually worked out in such a way that the amount of cream recommended for use contains about 20 mg of progesterone. The pessaries contain either 200 mg or 400 mg per dose, and the gel contains 400 mg per dose.

Another difference is that when the progesterone is administered transdermally it passes through the skin into the fat, from where it is released slowly into the bloodstream. The progesterone in the pessaries or gel is released rapidly, and is taken up through the mucosa into the bloodstream.

The high dose obtained from the pessaries and gel are suitable for use when you are taking high doses of additional oestrogens and need the progesterone to protect the lining of the uterus from becoming cancerous. They are also useful for treating very severe PMS and post-natal depression. The high doses do not seem to be so beneficial for the treatment of menopausal symptoms or osteoporosis.

ARE ALL NATURAL PROGESTERONE CREAMS THE SAME?

No, they are not. In order first for the natural progesterone to be absorbed from the cream it must be in a micronized form. If it is not, then absorption is very difficult – this is the problem with some of the 'home-made' creams. Another factor which can vary is the amount of natural progesterone in the cream. Often this is not stated on the label in actual figures; it is important that you find out from the manufacturer how much there is in the jar or tube you are using.

The amount you use each day can be calculated when you know the strength of the cream. The amount you use per day should be around 15–20 mg to be within normal physiological ranges.

Another thing to be aware of is what else is in the cream. There are a number of creams on the market that are called progesterone creams but contain other substances as well. Often these are phyto-oestrogens. There are also some creams which contain both progesterone and oestrogens. It is better to use the progesterone on its own initially, particularly if you are trying to solve symptoms of oestrogen dominance. If you do find that you need oestrogens or phyto-oestrogens, then it is usually better to have them in separate preparations so that you can adjust the progesterone and oestrogens separately to ensure that the ratio is correct for you.

WHAT ARE THE TOXICITY LEVELS AND SIDE-EFFECTS OF NATURAL PROGESTERONE?

There have not been any reported toxic effects of this natural hormone. The highest dose we are aware of is of a woman taking natural progesterone at the dose of 1,600 mg daily for 10 years, including during a pregnancy. This was in the form of suppositories. The trade name for these is Cyclogest, and they are frequently given in doses of 400 to 800 mg daily. According to Shire Pharmaceuticals, the drug company that makes them, they have only had three reported cases of possible visual side-effects, which ceased as soon as the Cyclogest was withdrawn.

If you are using natural progesterone in the form of a cream, it would be necessary to use half a tube per day to use as much as a woman's body naturally makes per day during pregnancy. The only side-effect that has been reported by people using the various available creams has been mild skin irritation. In all the cases we are aware of, this has been shown to be due to an allergic reaction to some other ingredient in the cream, not the progesterone.

CAN YOU OVERDOSE ON NATURAL PROGESTERONE?
It is difficult to overdose with natural progesterone but it could be done, especially if you are using an oral form, suppositories, or vaginal gel. These contain higher doses than the cream, and continued use of these forms can result in a high intake of progesterone. When using progesterone for the relief of symptoms the aim is to use a daily dose which is very close to the amount produced daily by the body when it is functioning normally. Over-dosage with the other forms of progesterone can cause drowsiness and visual disturbances. These symptoms disappear almost as soon as you stop using the progesterone.

HAVING COME OFF HRT, I DON'T FEEL THE NEED OF ANY EXTRA
OESTROGEN, BUT IS IT ALL RIGHT JUST TO TAKE PROGESTERONE?
Yes, progesterone can be used on its own without any additional oestrogen. When progesterone is being prescribed it is usually being used to counteract the effects on the body of an oestrogen dominance.

IS THERE A LIMIT ON HOW LONG I CAN USE NATURAL
PROGESTERONE?
There is no limit to the length of time you can use natural progesterone, provided that you are using it in a physiological

dosage (20–40 mg per day) and at the right time. This means on the correct days of your menstrual cycle, if you still have one, or having a few days without the progesterone each month if you are menopausal. The actual regime which you should follow will be advised by your practitioner.

However, it is important to realize that, like anything else, you should not continue to use a medication if you no longer need it. For this reason it is useful, after you have been using natural progesterone for a year or so and your symptoms have disappeared, to stop using the natural progesterone and see whether or not you still need to use it.

The only condition for which you probably would need to use natural progesterone long-term is osteoporosis, as it will continue to build up new bone regardless of your age. (See also Chapter 6.)

HOW LONG BEFORE I SEE ANY BENEFIT FROM USING NATURAL PROGESTERONE?

This will depend on why you are using it. If it is to correct osteoporosis, for example, you would not expect to see any benefits earlier than six months. If you are using it for PMS or other oestrogen-dominant symptoms you could see a result in two or three weeks, although it may take up to two months before you see any benefit. Everyone is different and therefore everyone responds differently to any treatment.

It is also important to realize that natural progesterone is not a cure-all for any and every symptom that seems to be related to a woman's hormone balance.

CAN YOU USE TOO MUCH NATURAL PROGESTERONE CREAM?

When using natural progesterone cream, you would have to rub in at least half a tube a day to produce the same amount as a woman's body naturally makes per day during pregnancy. As the instructions for use suggest that a tube should last 1–2 months, you can see it would be very hard to overdo it, but even if you did there would be no ill-effects, just rather a waste of the cream.

AFTER TWO MONTHS OF USE, MY SYMPTOMS HAVE NOT IMPROVED.
It is important to remember that natural progesterone is not a miracle drug and will not cure all health problems that occur in women. It may well be that the symptoms of which you complain are not due to lack of progesterone, or not caused by oestrogen dominance. Possibly you are in need of natural progesterone but are not using it in an appropriate way for your symptoms. No hard-and-fast rules can be given as to how long each individual will take to respond to any course of treatment, and natural progesterone is no exception. Hormones are powerful substances and should always be used under the guidance of a practitioner who is familiar not only with hormonal problems but also with the use of natural progesterone to treat them correctly.

I READ IN AN ARTICLE THAT HORMONES ARE CARCINOGENIC, AND I WORRY IF THERE IS ANY RISK?
Hormones in themselves are not carcinogenic (cancer-forming). They are substances produced by the endocrine glands of the body and have important roles to perform. If something happens to throw the balance of these hormones out then an excess of one or a lack of another can lead to cancer developing in certain organs.

Artificial hormones produced by the drug companies have chemical structures different from those of natural hormones even though they may have some of the same effects. It is the effect of these artificial hormones that can be cancer-forming.

Excess oestrogens, either as a result of imbalance in the body or as a result of being given extra oestrogen in the form of HRT, can cause cancer of the uterus and breast. This is because the effect of oestrogen on the cell receptors in the breast and endometrial tissue is to cause proliferation, and excessive cell proliferation leads to cancer.

Although virtually every paper published on the subject shows that there is a link between breast cancer and oestrogens, there still remains controversy as to how great this risk is and for how long a woman has to take oestrogen, or have oestrogen dominance, before the cancer occurs. This risk can be reduced dramatically if the oestrogen dominance is counteracted by natural progesterone. (See also Chapter 5.)

IF PROGESTERONE ENCOURAGES THE BREAKDOWN OF OLD CELLS AND THEIR REPLACEMENT WITH NEW YOUNG CELLS, WILL SUPPLEMENTATION WITH NATURAL PROGESTERONE KEEP ME YOUNG?

As far as we know there is nothing that will keep you young, and natural progesterone is no exception. In theory, supplementing with natural progesterone should help because of its effect on the turnover of cells and the way in which the death of old cells and their replacement with young cells is stimulated. This ought to make the skin look better, and possibly younger. So while there is no evidence to suggest that natural progesterone does keep you young, it should not be forgotten that progesterone creams were first sold in the US as cosmetic creams because of their apparent beneficial effect on the complexion. Certainly many women who use natural progesterone creams do comment on this benefit, but what effect it has on other tissues has not been reported.

I HAVE BEEN USING 200MG SUPPOSITORIES FOR THREE YEARS AND AM WORRIED THAT I AM TAKING TOO MUCH. MY DOCTOR WON'T PRESCRIBE A CREAM, SO WHAT CAN I DO?

You could always try cutting the suppository into halves, or quarters, and using these reduced amounts. Or use the suppository every other day. It is certainly not a good idea to stay on a high dose of this form of progesterone for too long, as it is the prolonged use of high-dose suppositories that can lead to side-effects.

MY DOCTOR PRESCRIBED PESSARIES FOR ME 10 YEARS AGO AND I AM STILL TAKING THEM. I AM WORRIED THAT THEY MIGHT AFFECT MY LONG-TERM HEALTH.
This is certainly exceptional, and you need to be vigilant for side-effects or changes in your condition. High doses would normally be given for short-term, critical conditions such as severe PMS, and are not expected to be a lifelong medication.

The problem with such high doses is that your own body's ability to produce progesterone is not stimulated, but overwhelmed; it is hard then for your own hormones to be in balance. You might want to discuss with your doctor changing to another form of progesterone if you are still in need of supplementing with it.

I CAN'T GET A PRESCRIPTION FOR PROGESTERONE CREAM, BUT I CAN GET ONE FOR CRINONE. CAN I USE THIS ON MY SKIN IN THE SAME WAY?
Crinone is designed as a vaginal gel, not for use on the skin. It is not really known how much you would absorb through the skin, and we would not suggest you try it.

IS CRINONE A NATURAL PROGESTERONE?
It is a natural form of progesterone, but has a slightly higher delivery than progesterone cream and will give you 400 mg per dose. Because it has a pump action it is more difficult to vary the dosage; it is generally indicated to be prescribed every other day, so this should even out the amount you receive.

WHAT TRIALS HAVE BEEN HELD USING PROGESTERONE?
A considerable number of trials have been held using progesterone. Details of these are available from the Natural

Progesterone Information Service (see Resources chapter). There are also trials on using natural progesterone creams being undertaken throughout the world. However, many of the benefits of progesterone are known from its reported use by many doctors over the past 20 to 25 years. It is interesting that during this time no adverse affects have been reported when progesterone is used in physiological doses. Some of the creams have produced skin reactions in some women, but this has been found to be caused by one of the other ingredients in the creams, not the progesterone itself.

WHAT TESTS ARE THERE FOR OESTROGEN AND PROGESTERONE, AND ARE THEY ACCURATE?

Women make several oestrogens in their body, the most important of which are oestradiol, oestrone and oestriol, and only one progesterone. These hormones can be measured in the blood and in the saliva. They can be measured daily throughout a cycle or on specific days. For a fuller description on hormone testing, see page 16.

Whether they are accurate is more difficult to answer. Blood tests your doctor will interpret for you, but with saliva tests you need really to be advised individually by a practitioner experienced in the use and interpretation of this particular form of testing. The laboratory will send you the results and compare them with so-called normal levels, but they will not be fully aware of your symptoms, and therefore the interpretation sent to you could be flawed.

With regard to the oestrogens, it should be remembered that the commonly used blood test only measures oestradiol, and that at or after menopause our oestrone levels rise as our oestradiol levels fall. If the oestrone is not measured as well, you may be diagnosed as abnormally low in oestrogen when in fact you are not.

WHY DO SOME PEOPLE SAY YOU SHOULD MEASURE PROGESTERONE
LEVELS IN BLOOD AND OTHERS SAY YOU SHOULD MEASURE IT IN
SALIVA? WHO IS CORRECT?

In fact both are correct. Progesterone can be found in both
saliva and in the blood. It is a matter of choice and availabil-
ity as to which method is chosen. Both have their uses.

MY DOCTOR SAYS MY HORMONE TESTS SHOW I AM MENOPAUSAL.
DOES THIS MEAN I AM LOW IN OESTROGEN OR PROGESTERONE?

In fact, oestrogens and progesterone are not the hormones
normally measured by doctors or even gynaecological consultants in diagnosing menopause. They measure the FSH
(Follicular Stimulating Hormone) and the LH (Leuteinizing
Hormone). These are hormones produced by the pituitary
which act on the ovary. If these are high it is assumed that
your ovary has stopped working and you are menopausal.
This is not always the case, however, and it is most important to measure the progesterone level, which can show
whether or not you are still ovulating. Ask your doctor to
re-test you on this basis to establish what your oestrogens
and progesterone levels really are before confirming that you
are menopausal.

I HAVE BEEN TOLD THAT THE NATURAL PROGESTERONE IN CREAMS
ACCUMULATES IN THE SKIN AND FAT AND DOES NOT ENTER THE
BODY.

If the progesterone is in a micronized form – as it is in the
creams – it will pass through the skin into the fat, be absorbed
and taken up by the fatty covering of the red blood cells and
transported to the progesterone receptors which exist in
many body tissues. When it reaches the tissues it can have
its effect.

If progesterone levels are measured with blood and saliva
tests after a woman has been using natural progesterone
in this form, then increased levels will be noted. The most

noticeable rise will be in the saliva, because the natural prog-esterone is carried in a fat-soluble form and is therefore not readily found in the blood serum.

AT A HEALTH SHOW I BOUGHT A PROGESTERONE CREAM FROM A
STAND. WAS THIS REALLY PROGESTERONE?
Progesterone cream can only be obtained in the UK on a doc-tor's prescription. It is not legal for any other practitioner other than a medically qualified doctor to prescribe it for you. It also may not be sold to you direct or over the counter in the UK.

In the list of ingredients on the tube or jar it will tell you what the contents are. If it specifically lists progesterone, then it is a cream containing natural progesterone and should only be obtained on medical prescription. If progesterone is not in the list of ingredients, then it is not a natural progesterone cream. A number of manufacturers are producing creams which contain wild yam or diosgenin, and their literature can suggest that the cream contains natural progesterone – but it does not. It is also important to remember that neither wild yam nor its active constituent diosgenin can be converted into any usable amounts of progesterone in the body.

WHAT'S THE DIFFERENCE BETWEEN WILD YAM AND PRO-GEST
CREAM?
There is a great deal of confusion about the difference between yam products and natural progesterone creams such as Pro-gest. They are completely different and therefore have different effects on the body. Mexican wild yam is a tuberous plant and is also classed as a herb. It has phyto-oestrogenic properties which enable it to be used to balance hormones. This means that it acts on oestrogen receptors, but its effect is not as strong as oestrogen. It also has a mild progestogenic effect and can be helpful in the treatment of certain menopausal symptoms and irregular periods.

HOW MUCH PROGESTERONE IS THERE IN WILD YAMS?
Mexican wild yam does not contain any progesterone and cannot be converted in the body to progesterone. Most progesterone creams contain natural progesterone made from a chemical which occurs naturally in wild yam called diosgenin. The progesterone is made in the laboratory from diosgenin extracted from wild yams, but the human body cannot duplicate this process and cannot convert diosgenin into natural progesterone by itself. This can only be done in the laboratory.

IF PROGESTERONE IS MADE IN THE LABORATORY, WHY IS IT CALLED NATURAL?
The progesterone which is made in the laboratory is identical in its chemical structure to progesterone made in the body. This is why it was first referred to as natural by Dr John Lee in his studies on the use of natural progesterone. He never intended it to imply that it came from a natural source, and regrets the confusion that has arisen over his perfectly legitimate use of the term.

I HAVE BEEN TOLD THAT JUST BECAUSE NATURAL PROGESTERONE HAS THE SAME CHEMICAL STRUCTURE AS PROGESTERONE MADE IN THE BODY, THAT DOES NOT MAKE IT NATURAL AND DOES NOT ENSURE IT HAS THE SAME EFFECT. THE COMPARISON MADE WAS WITH DIAMONDS, COAL AND THE GRAPHITE USED IN PENCILS ALL CARBON, BUT NOT ALL THE SAME.
While it is true that diamonds, the graphite in a pencil and coal are all carbon, the carbon atoms are arranged differently in the molecules of each of them. It is the molecular structure of the atoms, the way they are arranged, which determines what a substance is and how it behaves. The molecular structure of progesterone made in the body is identical to the molecular structure of natural progesterone made in the laboratory. As a result they are the same and behave in the same way in the body.

I CAN BUY PROGESTERONE CREAM FROM MY THERAPIST, SO WHY DO I NEED A PRESCRIPTION?

In the UK, natural progesterone is only available on prescription, so if you are in fact buying a genuine progesterone product then the person selling it to you is acting illegally. A clear guideline is that if you are buying a cream in the UK without a prescription, it cannot by law contain any progesterone. Creams containing progesterone can only be sold in the UK on prescription.

Confusion has arisen because it is perfectly legal to order natural progesterone products from outside the UK for your own use, and a number of suppliers do offer this facility. It is not legal, however, to order natural progesterone products to sell on to others.

MY DOCTOR SAYS THAT RESEARCH SHOWS THAT PROGESTERONE DOES NOT WORK. IS HE RIGHT?

Practitioners, and many of the women who use natural progesterone, will tell you it works from personal experience. In addition there is considerable research which shows that it works for specific conditions. Some reportedly adverse research has on investigation been shown to apply to the synthetic progestogens, not to natural progesterone.

There is no authenticated research that we are aware of that shows that natural progesterone does not work. However, some women who use it may find that it does not resolve the problems for which they started using it. This is because no medication will work for everybody. The best thing to do is to try it, because there is no evidence of any side-effects when it is used in physiological doses.

MY DOCTOR SAYS NATURAL PROGESTERONE IS UNTRIED AND HE WON'T PRESCRIBE IT FOR THAT REASON.

Natural progesterone has been used extensively in the USA and other parts of the world for over 20 years. A substantial body of research has also been carried out, and a considerable number of trials done. Details of these studies, and copies of the research papers, are obtainable from the Natural Progesterone Information Service (address on page 148).

Much of the knowledge of the effects of progesterone has been accumulated over the years by practitioners using it. There has been considerable difficulty in finding the funds for trials, which are very expensive, because progesterone is a natural substance and cannot therefore be patented, and thus does not attract the usual sources of funding, though hopefully this situation is now changing.

WHY CAN'T I GET IT ON THE NHS?

You can, but only at the discretion of your doctor. This will depend on his or her attitude and that of the practice and the local health authority. This should be easier when a licensed progesterone cream is available. Trials are currently being carried out on behalf of the Natural Medicine Company and it hopes to have a licensed cream available in the UK within a year or so.

IF NATURAL PROGESTERONE IS SO GOOD, WHY WON'T MY DOCTOR LET ME TRY IT?

The best person to explain this to you is your doctor. Ask him or her to explain to you fully the reason for this decision. There are many possible reasons. It may relate to his or her practice or to health authority policy or funding. It may be that your doctor does not know much about progesterone and is therefore acting correctly in not allowing you to use it. It is not ethical for doctors to prescribe a drug with which they are unfamiliar, because they will not be able to give you the advice and care you need. It may be that your doctor does not consider it to be appropriate for your condition. The thing to do is ask; if the problem is lack of information, suggest to your doctor that he or she contact some of the distributors and manufacturers of the available products, or write to the Natural Progesterone Information Service. You will find the relevant addresses on page 148 .

CAN I MAKE MY OWN NATURAL PROGESTERONE CREAM BY MELTING A PROGESTERONE SUPPOSITORY INTO A CREAM BASE?

The manufacturers of Cyclogest have made it quite clear that this is definitely *not* a good idea. This is for several reasons. First, this form of progesterone is designed for internal use and is not going to be absorbed well into the skin, so you will not get any benefit from it. Secondly, any form of do-it-yourself cream is an unknown quantity. You will not know how much progesterone it will contain, how active that progesterone will be, how stable it will be, or if it will actually have any effect at all. Also, whatever is used as a base will also have an effect depending on what it contains in the way of ingredients, so again you cannot rely on the outcome.

WILL DOCTORS BE TOLD OF THE RESULTS OF NATURAL PROGESTERONE TRIALS SO THEY CAN BE MORE CONVINCED TO PRESCRIBE IT?

The results of a considerable number of trials on natural progesterone, and research papers on these trials, are already available to anyone who wants them. Your doctor (or you yourself) need only contact the Natural Progesterone Information Service.

However, the fact that your doctor may have this information does not always result in his or her being convinced one way or the other. If a doctor wishes to be convinced of the validity of natural progesterone there is plenty of research material available, but in fact this is not necessary. All a doctor has to do is call to mind the physiology of progesterone, or look it up in any physiology textbook.

CHAPTER 3

The Fertile Years

THE FERTILE YEARS – INTRODUCTION

It would seem that nature intended women after puberty to spend a great deal of our time either pregnant or breastfeeding. Indeed, until comparatively recent times this was the role or fate of most women. Now things are rather different; many women will not have any pregnancies at all, and those who have children will not often have more than three or four.

As a result of this change in a woman's life pattern, we experience many more menstrual cycles than nature intended. The interesting thing in relation to this is that women do not stop menstruating earlier than they did a generation or so ago. In fact they often continue to ovulate for a longer time, so there is clearly no shortage of follicles and eggs. What will be lacking, however, is the respite from ovulation. This means that we spend more of our lives exposed to high oestrogen levels and less of our lives exposed to the protective effects of progesterone. This may be why such problems as osteoporosis, PMS, endometriosis, polycystic disease of the ovaries and breast cancer are so common.

Because of the large number of menstrual cycles which we experience as a result of fewer pregnancies than nature intended, few women pass through their menstrual phase of life without some problems. Often these problems are transient, but sometimes we are not so fortunate.

The pattern of a woman's hormonal life and monthly cycle is explained in the first chapter; here we are going to look in more detail at what can go wrong during a woman's fertile years – those between puberty and menopause.

If oestrogen and progesterone remain in balance, then the monthly cycle will continue with few problems. However, hormone balance these days is the exception rather than the rule for the majority of women, for a variety of reasons. A major one is stress caused by illness, injury, work pressures and emotional changes – which can all work to upset this balance.

This disturbance from stress is dealt with in the body by the *hypothalamus*. The hypothalamus is an area of the brain which controls not only our whole hormone balance but the way the body deals with stress, hunger, fluid balance, temperature control and other basic bodily functions. A change in any one of these systems can easily affect another part of the body. It is therefore easy to see how lifestyle, stress, diet, weight loss and gain, pollution and drugs can all affect hormone balance and lead to problems.

Many of the problems which occur and relate to the menstrual cycle may be helped by supplementing with natural progesterone.

THE FERTILE YEARS:
THE MENSTRUAL CYCLE

Puberty

At puberty the hormonal cycle starts. At first this is unlikely to be regular. Some young women have a period and then several months will pass before they have another. This is not a matter for concern, and most settle down eventually to a regular monthly cycle. It is important to remember that regular does not necessarily mean every 28 days. A 28 day menstrual cycle is an average; many women have regular cycles of 24 days or 30 days. It does not matter that we are all different.

It is difficult to say at what age a young girl should start her periods. Some will start as young as 13 or even as early as 9 or 10, while still others will not start until 19 or 20. Often this will follow a family pattern, and provided the girl is otherwise fit and well, the actual age is not important. If periods have not started by the age of 20 then it would be sensible to have the matter investigated, especially if there are no other signs of developing maturity, as there may be a medical problem that requires attention.

Menstrual Problems

Once the monthly cycle has started, the main problems which may be encountered are:

- painful periods
- heavy periods
- irregular periods
- symptoms of pre-menstrual stress
- periods stopping after becoming established.

All of these problems can relate to an imbalance of the oestrogens and progesterone being secreted at different phases of the cycle, and may be treatable with the supplementary use of natural progesterone.

These imbalances may be the result of dietary changes such as trying to lose weight, or excessive exercise as a result of sport, dance or gymnastic training. Stress can also affect the hormone balance in young women, whether it is caused by personal or family problems or the stress of studying to pass examinations. Although natural progesterone may be helpful, it is very important to first deal with the cause of the stress.

The Pill

Any young girl whose cycle is not well established should avoid going on the contraceptive pill. It is often prescribed to regulate the periods, and while it will certainly cause the bleed to occur at 28-day intervals this is not solving the problem. In fact it can often lead to enormous difficulty in establishing a cycle when the Pill is stopped, because a normal hormone balance has never been allowed to develop in the first place.

Menstrual Difficulties Once the Cycle Is Established

These can range from simple discomfort to serious gynaecological conditions which may require medical intervention. They include PMS, heavy bleeding, endometriosis, anovulatory cycles, or cervical or endometrial cancers. The root of the majority of them, however, can be traced to an excess of oestrogen over progesterone in the body.

This is known as oestrogen dominance. Symptoms include:

- water retention
- breast swelling and pain
- fibrocystic breasts
- premenstrual mood swings
- depression
- loss of libido
- heavy or irregular periods
- uterine fibroids
- craving for sweets
- weight gain, fat deposits on hips and thighs
- increased risk of breast, cervical and endometrial cancers.

See also the lists on page 4–6.

The Fertile Years – Menstrual Cycle: Questions and Answers

I HAVE HEARD THAT IF I USE NATURAL PROGESTERONE EARLIER THAN DAY 12 IN MY CYCLE I WILL NOT OVULATE. IS THIS TRUE?

Progesterone is normally secreted by the ovary after ovulation. This progesterone is produced by the follicle which has ovulated. As the level of progesterone rises, it has an effect on the pituitary, causing the pituitary to slow down the production of Leuteinizing Hormone – the hormone that stimulates follicles to rupture and thus causes ovulation. However, it seems that the mechanism involved in ovulation is more complex than this, and suppressing ovulation requires more than a high level of progesterone. It is unlikely that using progesterone before day 12 in your cycle would stop you from ovulating, and you certainly could not rely on using natural progesterone in this way as a method of contraception. If you are actually trying to get pregnant, you should only use progesterone cream after ovulation.

MY CONSULTANT HAS SUGGESTED A COIL CONTAINING
PROGESTERONE TO CONTROL MY HEAVY PERIODS – IS THIS A
GOOD IDEA?

The coil or intrauterine device that your consultant has suggested is probably the Mirena Coil. It is a common misconception, but this coil does *not* contain progesterone. It contains levonorgestrel, which is a progestogen, an artificial hormone that has some progesterone-like effects on the uterus. It may well help to control your heavy periods, but there has not been very much research done on it as it has only been available a few years and the long-term effects are not known. What we *do* know are that progestogens only mimic the action of progesterone and often have side-effects which can be very unpleasant. Those listed for the Mirena coil are:

- altered menstrual pattern
- headaches
- abdominal pain
- backache
- skin disorders
- breast tenderness
- vaginitis
- mood changes
- nausea
- fluid retention
- ovarian cysts
- pelvic inflammatory disease.

Side-effects do vary from one person to another. You may get none at all, only slight effects, or any of the above listed. As with all drugs, it is sensible to consider very carefully whether the listed side-effects are worth the possible benefits. It would certainly be worth asking your consultant to give you a trial period on natural progesterone first before undertaking the implantation of the Mirena Coil.

ON HRT I HAD NORMAL MONTHLY PERIODS, BUT WITH NATURAL
PROGESTERONE THEY HAVE STOPPED COMPLETELY. IS THIS USUAL?

Some women do find that HRT causes a bleed to happen
when the body may not have continued to do so on its own. If
that is the case, then when you stop taking the HRT this artificially-induced bleeding will also stop. There are also other
factors to consider as well. Ask your doctor to arrange for an
ultrasound scan of your uterus so that you can tell whether
or not the endometrium is building up. If it isn't, then there
is no need to worry because no bleeding should be happening.
If it is building up, however, then it must be dispersed and it
may be that you need to increase the amount of progesterone
you are taking to ensure that you do get a monthly bleed.

MY PROBLEM IS THAT MY PERIODS WILL NOT STOP. MY DOCTOR
HAS PRESCRIBED NORETHISTERONE WHICH HAS STOPPED THE
BLEEDING, BUT MAKES ME FEEL TERRIBLE. CAN I DO ANYTHING
ELSE?

This condition is known as dysfunctional uterine bleeding
and it is caused by oestrogen dominance. In theory this
should be controllable with natural progesterone because it
will help balance the unopposed oestrogens that are causing
the problem, but unfortunately once this condition gets
established it needs very strong measures to deal with the
bleeding. Chemical hormones like norethisterone are sometimes the only way to stop this very heavy continuous bleeding as the first course of treatment.

However, once the bleeding is under control, it is possible
– and indeed desirable – to change over to natural progesterone. You will need the help of a practitioner to do this
because the dosage of natural progesterone will be high, and
you need to be monitored and the dose adjusted as you are
taking it. If the bleeding gets out of control again you may
have to revert to norethisterone for a short time, but after a
few months it ought to be possible to control the bleeding

with natural progesterone alone. Also, of course, you will be helping to bring your body back to a situation where the oestrogen is not dominant and this distressing bleeding should not occur.

I HAVE VERY HEAVY AND PROLONGED PERIODS AND MY DOCTOR HAS SUGGESTED A D & C PROCEDURE. CAN I AVOID THIS?

If your periods are heavy and prolonged then you are oestrogen dominant, and the previous answer may also be helpful for you. The purpose of a D & C (dilatation and currettage – sometimes also referred to as a 'scrape') is to remove the thick lining of the womb which has been built up by the oestrogens and is not shed completely every month. Each month this lining continues to be built up and the amount of bleeding and length of your period seems to increase along with it.

Yes, natural progesterone will help to reduce the problem with your periods, and if the build-up is not too great it is also possible that you can avoid having a D & C. Ask your doctor if you can try natural progesterone for a few months and see if this will help. It may be, however, that the build-up is too great, in which case you might be better advised to have the D & C and make sure you then start using natural progesterone so that the oestrogen dominance does not recur.

I HAVE SOME SPOTTING OF BLOOD MID-CYCLE. WOULD NATURAL PROGESTERONE HELP?

Mid-cycle spotting is not a serious problem and usually relates to ovulation. It does not seem to relate to oestrogen dominance and it is probable that natural progesterone would not make any difference to it.

THROUGHOUT THE MONTH I GET SOME SPOTTING. IT IS NOT TO A REGULAR PATTERN BUT IT IS FAIRLY FREQUENT, AND I WONDERED IF I WAS PROGESTERONE DEFICIENT?

Spotting that occurs throughout a cycle, and is not related just to the few days around ovulation, is a symptom of oestrogen dominance. Try using natural progesterone for a few months, but if the spotting continues then it *must* be investigated further by your doctor. This type of bleeding can be an early sign of ovarian problems, endometrial cancer and cervical abnormalities such as erosion or cancer of the cervix.

COULD I USE NATURAL PROGESTERONE TO POSTPONE MY PERIOD BEFORE MY WEDDING?

No, it is not really a viable option. Progesterone is produced naturally by the corpus luteum after ovulation. This has the effect of maturing the lining of the uterus to prepare it for a pregnancy. If the egg is not fertilized, the levels of progesterone drop dramatically and menstruation occurs. If the egg is fertilized, the levels of progesterone remain high and the lining of the uterus is not shed. It seems as if the effect of progesterone at this time is to prevent menstruation, and therefore that the use of natural progesterone supplementation in this way would postpone menstruation.

However, using natural progesterone does *not* seem to be effective in postponing menstruation when a pregnancy has not occurred. It may be that the levels of progesterone need to be very high, but it seems more likely that other hormonal changes, such as the secretion of Human Chorionic Gonadotrophin by the fertilized egg, are also involved. For these reasons you could not rely on progesterone to postpone your period.

WHAT EXACTLY ARE FIBROIDS, AND HOW WOULD I KNOW IF
I HAD ANY?
Fibroids are caused by unopposed oestrogen and are benign
uterine tumours made up of muscle and fibrous tissue. They
can be very small – the size of a pea – to very large, more like
a grapefruit, but are rarely painful. Fibroids usually need to
be diagnosed by pelvic examination and scan. Unfortunately
symptoms of them aren't very visible, but most commonly
women experience very heavy bleeding and a greater fre-
quency of urinating. You may also find it helpful to read
the questions on fibroids in the pre-menopause section in
Chapter 4 (page 73).

HOW EFFECTIVE IS NATURAL PROGESTERONE IN INHIBITING
AND REDUCING UTERINE FIBROIDS?
Uterine fibroids are an indication that the body is oestrogen
dominant. When a woman enters menopause her oestrogen
levels fall, and this is why fibroids tend to regress naturally
during that time. If natural progesterone is used to try to correct the oestrogen dominance in someone who has fibroids,
it may stop the fibroids from growing any bigger. However,
unless the uterine fibroids are small it is unlikely that they
will disappear altogether. It is sometimes the case that the
heavy bleeding often associated with uterine fibroids is
reduced, and for many women this is a major help in dealing
with the situation. This reduction in bleeding may be due
to the fact that the body is less oestrogen-dominant and as a
result of this the uterine lining that is built up during the
cycle is less thick.

MY MOTHER AND SISTERS BOTH SUFFER FROM FIBROIDS. I DON'T
HAVE ANY, BUT IF I TAKE NATURAL PROGESTERONE WILL IT
PREVENT ME GETTING THEM?
Fibroids are one of the most common problems for peri-
menopausal women, but there is no specific evidence to

show that the use of natural progesterone will prevent them occurring in the first place. However, as they are a condition of oestrogen dominance you would be sensible to monitor yourself for symptoms of this and take natural progesterone if appropriate.

I AM BEING RECOMMENDED TO HAVE A HYSTERECTOMY FOR VERY LARGE FIBROIDS WHICH CAUSE A LOT OF BLEEDING. I HAVE BEEN GIVEN HRT TO TRY AND CONTROL THEM, BUT WOULD NATURAL PROGESTERONE BE HELPFUL AS WELL?

It is a very big step to have a hysterectomy simply to remove fibroids. Unless they are life-threatening, which is very rare, you are undertaking major surgery which can have very serious long-term consequences.

Fibroids are a result of unopposed oestrogen. Unfortunately the treatment often involves giving more oestrogen, as in HRT, and then the fibroids get worse. The best plan would be to stop taking oestrogen and supplement with natural progesterone to prevent the fibroids getting larger. At menopause, when your oestrogen levels drop, your fibroids will shrink naturally. In addition to natural progesterone, herbal medicine, acupuncture and homoeopathy can all offer some assistance with the problem of heavy bleeding.

I HAVE BEEN GIVEN DANOL TO REDUCE MY FIBROIDS PRIOR TO SURGERY. MY DOCTOR SAYS I CAN'T USE NATURAL PROGESTERONE AS WELL. WHY EVER NOT?

Danol (generic name danazol) is a drug with a wide range of conflicting hormonal effects and a number of side-effects. It is often used quite successfully for a short time before surgery for fibroids because it seems to reduce their size and vascularity and this makes the surgery easier.

It would be pointless to use natural progesterone at the same time as Danol because danazol is such a potent drug that it would not allow the natural progesterone to have any

practical effect, and in fact taking hormones is contraindicated when also taking Danol. It is also unlikely that using
natural progesterone instead of Danol prior to surgery would
reduce the vascularity or size of the fibroids. However it may
reduce the severity of the symptoms from the fibroids, such
as pain and heavy bleeding, and it may also prevent them
from growing.

These benefits may be enough to make surgery unnecessary, so talk to your consultant about using natural progesterone instead of a powerful drug like Danol.

IS IT NECESSARY TO TAKE DANOL BEFORE A HYSTERECTOMY?

The previous question will partly answer your question. If
your consultant wants you to take Danol before surgery,
ask him or her why. If it is to reduce the size of fibroids,
reduce vascularity of the uterus or reduce the extent of your
endometriosis in order to make the surgery easier and therefore safer, you should probably do as he or she suggests.

However, it is important that you do not take Danol
longer than about six months, and that you are not on any
drugs that are contraindicated when prescribed Danol. These
include some anti-convulsants, insulin, some anti-coagulants,
other hormones and alcohol. The side-effects of Danol are
numerous and include menstrual disturbances, weight gain,
skin rashes, cardio-vascular disturbances such as raised blood
pressure and palpitations, and visual disturbances; Danol can
also bring on a migraine attack in those already susceptible.
It is sensible if a drug like Danol is recommended by a consultant who is probably only concerned with your gynaecological problems, and not familiar with your full medical
history, that you discuss it in detail with your doctor. They
should be able to help you, and together you can discuss if
Danol really is suitable for you, before you go back to see
your consultant.

I AM TAKING DANOL BEFORE MY MYOMECTOMY, BUT WANT TO
USE NATURAL PROGESTERONE AS WELL. HOW DO I DO THIS?
What would be most effective would be to take the natural
progesterone *after* you have had the surgery and when your
own menstrual cycle is re-established. The main reason to do
this is to prevent oestrogen dominance. You will want to prevent the possible development of further fibroids if you have
a myomectomy and the further effects of oestrogen dominance on the body as a whole.

I AM IN MY LATE TWENTIES AND MY PERIODS HAVE BECOME
SLIGHTLY IRREGULAR. I HAVE ALSO STARTED TO HAVE A PROBLEM
WITH INCREASED FACIAL HAIR. SHOULD I USE NATURAL
PROGESTERONE?
Your description of irregular periods and development of
facial hair suggests that you may be suffering from the condition known as polycystic disease of the ovaries. Your doctor
should be able to confirm or disprove this diagnosis by
arranging a hormone test and a pelvic ultrasound scan.

If you do have this condition you should certainly benefit
from supplementation with natural progesterone. When you
have polycystic ovaries, for some reason (which is not fully
understood) ovulation does not occur. As a result, the developing follicles in the ovary remain as cysts, and – because
ovulation has not occurred – no corpus luteum forms and no
progesterone is made. If you supplement with natural progesterone this helps to restore the balance.

Also there is often a rise of testosterone in this condition,
and when the oestrogen/progesterone balance is restored the
testosterone levels seem to drop back to normal.

CAN NATURAL PROGESTERONE HELP WITH POLYCYSTIC DISEASE
OF THE OVARY?
The term polycystic disease of the ovary refers to a whole
group of disorders with considerable differences in their

clinical and hormonal picture. They all show to some degree a failure to ovulate, though the cause of this is not clear. Symptoms can include irregular periods or lack of menstruation, obesity and increased amounts of facial or body hair. Hormonal studies often show disturbed body levels including raised oestrogen, raised Leuteinizing Hormone and raised testosterone, with low Follicular Stimulating Hormone and low progesterone. Patients who exhibit these symptoms are usually followed up with pelvic ultrasound scanning; if polycystic disease is present the scan will reveal many small cysts on the ovaries.

There is no ideal therapy for this condition. Orthodox medicine frequently advises taking the contraceptive pill, but this is not a cure.

Natural progesterone has been used to treat polycystic ovaries and may help to resolve the condition by having an effect on the feedback mechanism between the ovary and the pituitary. The natural progesterone may be supplemented on a continuous basis for three to four months to 'rest' the ovary. Then it can be used for two weeks, followed by a break for two weeks. This mimics the normal secretion of progesterone in the body and may regulate the ovary-pituitary feedback mechanism. This dosage regime will need to be adjusted as you go along, especially if you do not know what your normal cycle is.

Patients have been helped by supplementing with natural progesterone, but because it is a complex condition you should seek the help of a practitioner who is familiar with the use of natural hormones for this condition.

I WANT TO USE NATURAL PROGESTERONE FOR MY ENDOMETRIOSIS, BUT MY CONSULTANT SAYS IT WON'T HELP.
Endometriosis is a condition in which endometrial tissue – that is, tissue which normally lines the uterus, is found in areas where it should not be. It can be on the ovary, fallopian

tubes, in the uterine muscle and on the outside of any intra-abdominal organ. These pieces of endometrium respond to the hormonal changes each month in the same way as the lining of the uterus. As a result, these pieces of tissue proliferate, swell and bleed, and in doing so cause considerable pain and other problems such as adhesions, bowel obstruction and blockage of the fallopian tubes.

The cause of endometriosis is not known, and treatment by orthodox methods is difficult, often has unpleasant side-effects and sometimes doesn't even work. Because the endometrial tissue responds to hormones in the same way as the lining of the uterus, it proliferates under the effect of oestrogen. This proliferation can be stopped by the use of progesterone. What is critical is to get the right amount of progesterone at the right time in your cycle, and this needs to be worked out for you by a practitioner familiar with the use of progesterone. No clinical trials in relation to this specific use of progesterone have been done at the time of writing, but many women have reported dramatic results and a great improvement in their condition.

You may also find it helpful to read the question on endometrial cancer in Chapter 5 (page 109).

I AM 42 AND STILL HAVING PERIODS, THOUGH THESE HAVE BECOME VERY IRREGULAR. I HAVE BECOME VERY DEPRESSED AND TIRED AND WONDERED IF NATURAL PROGESTERONE MIGHT MAKE A DIFFERENCE?
Even though you are still having periods it is possible that you may not be ovulating, or if you are ovulating that you are not having a full progesterone surge in the second half of your cycle. When oestrogen is not balanced by progesterone, two of the effects of this can be depression and tiredness, and certainly progesterone would be a positive start to treating those symptoms.

You should start the cream on day seven of your cycle and

use it either until your period starts or you reach day 27, then stop. If you have a period, repeat the regime. If no period arrives, start the cream again after seven days. You could also be a bit anaemic, so perhaps try a herbal tonic containing some easily-absorbed iron. Many women find this very helpful.

Also well-known for its ability to lift depression is the herb hypericum, or St John's Wort. This is available in tablets from most health stores and major pharmacists, and if you have a local herbalist they may make you an individual tincture with hypericum and Kava Kava, which is also often suggested for depression.

MY DOCTOR WANTS TO GIVE ME ANTIDEPRESSANTS BUT I THINK MY SYMPTOMS ARE HORMONAL AS THEY ARE RELATED TO MY MENSTRUAL CYCLE. HOW CAN I CONVINCE HER?

If you believe your symptoms are hormonal in origin you are probably correct. Convincing your doctor, however, may not be so easy. You should keep a diary of your symptoms and show how they relate to your menstrual cycle. This may help to prove your point. If not, then remind her of the fact that it is well recognized, as a result of work done by Dr Katharina Dalton, that a lack of progesterone can cause depression in the premenstrual phase. Also remind her that post-natal depression is due to a drop in progesterone after delivery. If this doesn't work, then ask for a 'trial run' using progesterone for two or three months to see what happens. If she will still not prescribe it for you, ask if she would object if you consulted a doctor familiar with the use of natural progesterone prescribing. The Natural Progesterone Information Service can provide you with a list (address on page 148).

SINCE MY PERIODS BECAME IRREGULAR TWO YEARS AGO, I HAVE
NOTICED MY HAIR FALLING OUT. COULD NATURAL PROGESTERONE
HELP?

It is possible that your hair loss relates to your hormone
imbalance. You will have noticed that many women have
beautiful hair when they are pregnant, a time when progesterone levels are very high. It could well be worthwhile supplementing with some natural progesterone and seeing what
happens.

Do remember that with hair loss you must not expect
a quick response. You may notice less hair falling out after
three months' use, but you will not see an increased growth
of new hair before about six months. It is also important to
visit a trichologist to make sure that you do not have a scalp
problem which could be the cause of the hair loss. Also ask
your doctor to check your iron and ferritin levels, as if these
are low it can also lead to loss of hair. (See Resources page 154.)

I SUFFER FROM EPILEPTIC FITS BUT THESE ONLY OCCUR
DURING THE DAYS JUST BEFORE MY PERIOD. COULD NATURAL
PROGESTERONE HELP?

It has been shown that epileptic attacks which only occur
during the premenstrual period will sometimes respond to
supplementation with natural progesterone. This can often
be so effective that the need for taking other anti-epileptic
drugs can be removed. If you want to try this it is important
to discuss it with, and have the co-operation of, your own
doctor.

I THINK I MAY HAVE PMS, BUT HOW CAN I BE SURE?

There are so many different symptoms that can be ascribed
to PMS, or Premenstrual Syndrome, that it can often be
difficult to be certain if any specific one is related to this
condition. Certainly Dr John Lee mentions over a hundred
symptoms in his experience – though happily no one woman

will experience more than a few of these at any one time. It is certainly a widespread condition today, and it's estimated that around 60 to 80 per cent of all menstruating women between the ages of 20 and 50 do get regular symptoms of PMS. It's much more common in industrial and technologically advanced countries, and contributory factors are poor diet, high stress levels, synthetic hormone use, oestrogen-dominance symptoms and the role played by xeno-oestrogens and pollutants. This is a checklist of some of the most common symptoms which women report (you may have just one or several of them):

breast tenderness
breast swelling
depression
mood swings
bloating
weight gain
exhaustion
loss of libido
headaches
irritability/anger.

These symptoms can usually be successfully treated with short-term supplementation with natural progesterone to restore the hormone balance.

I HAVE TRIED SO MANY THINGS FOR MY PMS. WHY SHOULD NATURAL PROGESTERONE BE ANY DIFFERENT?
First you must understand what is causing your PMS. You have symptoms caused by an excess of oestrogen in relation to the progesterone in your body, and although other treatments may help to alleviate this imbalance it is really only through supplementation with the 'missing' hormone that you can restore your body to its normal state. Of course other

factors are important – diet, for instance is vital when treating PMS – but if you are basically not producing enough progesterone, as many young women do not these days, then only the natural hormone progesterone will restore that balance.

MY PMS IS VERY SEVERE. MY DOCTOR HAS SUGGESTED ORAL
PROGESTERONE, RATHER THAN THE CREAM. WHAT IS THE
DIFFERENCE?
It's really a difference in absorption and how the body deals with processing the progesterone. Oral progesterone requires 5–8 times the daily dose to obtain the same results as you would get by using a progesterone cream applied to the skin. Approximately 80 per cent of oral progesterone is intercepted by the liver and excreted in the bile. Additionally, oral progesterone will produce a sharp rise in serum progesterone levels followed by a rapid drop in serum levels within several hours. For this reason alone a transdermal cream is recommended because it will give you more consistent and slower release into the bloodstream, and this helps the body utilize the progesterone more effectively.

The drawback to natural progesterone creams, however, is that it is impossible to take very high doses. If your PMS is very severe then it may be that oral supplementation, or indeed progesterone pessaries, may be the best way to quickly bring it under control. However, once you have done that it would be advisable to switch to the cream so you are then getting a more physiological dose – that is, one that your own body will recognize as normal.

I WOULD LIKE TO TRY NATURAL PROGESTERONE, BUT AS I HAVE
IRRITABLE BOWEL SYNDROME I WONDER IF IT WOULD AFFECT IT?
Irritable Bowel Syndrome varies from person to person. If you find that your symptoms are worse during the time leading up to your period then it is certainly possible that using natural progesterone could help. Progesterone is a muscle

relaxant, and if you have spasm associated with oestrogen dominance then progesterone should help to relax it.

I HAVE MS AND HAVE TO BE CAREFUL WHAT MEDICATION I TAKE. COULD NATURAL PROGESTERONE HAVE ANY HARMFUL EFFECT?
It is unlikely that natural progesterone could have any harmful effects, especially if you use it in the physiological dose recommended: 20 to 40 mg per day. It is in fact possible that progesterone could have a beneficial effect on MS symptoms, although no scientific studies have been done on this. It is known that progesterone is involved in the synthesis of myelin sheaths. These are the sheaths which protect the peripheral nerves, and it is thought that a deficiency of myelin is a factor in the progression of MS. If a substance helps in the synthesis of these sheaths it is possible that it could help to control the progression of MS. It must be stressed that there are at present no clinical studies to support this idea.

THE FERTILE YEARS: THE BREASTS

The breasts are in fact a pair of glands; their main function is to provide milk for a newborn child. They are what is known as a secondary sex characteristic. In other words, they indicate femaleness but are not present when a female child is born. They are very important to a woman's concept of her femininity, a point often forgotten when surgery on them is suggested. Normally a woman only has two breasts but it is not uncommon for women to have extra nipples. These occur along the milk line, which extends from under the armpit, towards the natural position for a nipple, and then down to the mid-groin. When women have these extra nipples it is rare – though not unknown – for additional breasts to develop at the site of the extra nipples.

The breasts start to develop at the beginning of puberty, often quite some time before menstruation itself starts. This development is the result of stimulation by the increasing levels of oestrogens in the body. There are two main tissues which make up a breast: fatty tissue and glandular tissue. It is useful to remember that when in the inactive state, before breastfeeding, most of the breast tissue is fat. The size of a woman's breasts is no indicator of her ability to produce milk. During a pregnancy the high levels of oestrogens and progesterone cause the glandular tissue of the breast to develop and prepare itself for lactation. As soon as the baby is born the pituitary secretes a hormone called prolactin which stimulates lactation. Once a baby starts to feed, the action of sucking on the breasts stimulates lactation and encourages the release of prolactin by the pituitary.

The changing levels of oestrogens and progesterone which occur during a normal monthly cycle also affect the breast. After ovulation the increasing level of oestrogens cause the breasts to become swollen and often they become tender. This effect disappears as soon as the period starts. If a situation of oestrogen dominance exists, then this stimulation of the breast tissue by oestrogens becomes more marked. The breasts can become very engorged and painful prior to a period and may form cysts, lumps or cancers. It is now generally accepted that all breast cancers are either caused or aggravated by excess oestrogens. Where symptoms suggesting oestrogen dominance exist the use of natural progesterone will usually relieve the problem.

The Fertile Years – The Breasts: Questions and Answers

EVERY MONTH BEFORE MY PERIOD MY BREASTS ARE LUMPY
AND PAINFUL. WHAT CAN I DO?
Technically, you have fibrocystic breasts – one of the classic
signs of oestrogen dominance. They can be treated with natural progesterone (see usage guide on page 17 - 18), and generally respond fairly quickly to treatment. Some women also
find that supplementing with vitamin E, magnesium and vitamin B_6 can also be helpful.

MY BREASTS GET TENDER AND SWOLLEN EVERY MONTH. WILL
NATURAL PROGESTERONE HELP WITH THIS?
Oestrogen is the factor that is causing this problem, and it is
probably not being balanced with sufficient progesterone.
Also, although we might not normally associate fluid retention with the breasts, they can also be prone to this, making
them swell and be very tender. Supplementation with natural progesterone for three weeks out of four in your cycle
could help to restore the oestrogen-to-progesterone balance
and solve the problem with your breasts. Don't expect it
to be cured straight away; sometimes when you start taking
progesterone for this condition the breast tenderness initially becomes worse before getting better.

CAN I USE NATURAL PROGESTERONE IF I AM BREASTFEEDING?
It is very unlikely that you would need to take progesterone
at that time, because when a woman is breastfeeding she
produces high levels of a hormone called prolactin. One of the
effects of prolactin, other than milk production, is to lower
oestrogen levels in the body. It is therefore extremely
unlikely that any symptoms of oestrogen dominance would
exist, so you would not need to take any additional progesterone.

HRT GAVE ME PAINFUL BREASTS. WILL NATURAL PROGESTERONE DO
THIS AS WELL?

HRT gave you painful breasts because the amount of oestrogen it contained was too high for you. The oestrogen had a
stimulating effect upon the breasts and this was not balanced
by having natural progesterone. HRT contains artificial
progestogens, which do not have the same balancing effect as
the natural hormone; nor do progestogens have any protective effect on the breast. Taking natural progesterone does
not stimulate the oestrogen receptors and you therefore
should not experience painful breasts as a result of taking it,
in fact quite the reverse.

THE FERTILE YEARS: FERTILITY

AND INFERTILITY

An Introduction

It is a common fallacy that all a woman has to do to become
pregnant is to stop using contraception. For a lucky minority
who are ready to start their families this may indeed be the
case, but for many other women and their partners timing is
all-important, with both having careers. Postponing a family
until the woman is in her late thirties is an option that is
occurring more and more frequently. Unfortunately when
these couples do come to start a family it is not as simple as
making the decision and giving up contraception. Some
women find at this stage that conception is not automatic, or
easy, and indeed it can be a very difficult and stressful time.

Factors for a Successful Conception

For a pregnancy to occur the body needs a very specific sequence of events to take place, and all of them in the right order, so timing is also a crucial factor.

First the woman needs to produce a healthy egg, which must meet with healthy sperm, and the woman also needs to ovulate. As the egg is produced a day or so prior to it reaching the point in the fallopian tubes where it can meet with the sperm, you can see that it has to be healthy so that it will survive long enough to be fertilized. Then it actually has to be fertilized by the sperm and the newly-fertilized embryo must be able to survive its journey down the fallopian tube to the uterus. Even then, other factors are still coming into play. When the embryo reaches the uterus the endometrium or lining of the uterus must be in a mature and stable state so that implantation can occur and a placenta form. Apart from the actual development of the egg and ovulation itself, for all these stages to succeed they require the presence of progesterone.

The progesterone needed is produced by the ovary from the corpus luteum, which is the remains of the follicle after ovulation. Normally when a woman ovulates, sufficient progesterone will be produced by the corpus luteum to ensure that the egg survives long enough to be fertilized. After fertilization has occurred an embryo is formed. The embryo then secretes a hormone known as Human Chorionic Gonadotrophin. This hormone reaches the corpus luteum and stimulates it to produce large quantities of progesterone. This ensures the survival of the embryo until it has safely implanted itself in the uterus and a placenta has formed. It is that placenta which takes over the job of making progesterone throughout the pregnancy. Any failure in the production of progesterone at any point in this story can result in a miscarriage. Progesterone, as its name tells us, is the hormone 'for gestation'; in other words it is the pregnancy hormone.

What Can Go Wrong

When investigating a woman who has not become pregnant after trying for some time, it is a standard procedure to measure her progesterone levels on day 20 (if she has a 28-day cycle) to establish whether or not she has ovulated. A rise of progesterone to a specific level indicates that this has happened. It is then often assumed that because she is producing progesterone at this point in her cycle she will go on producing sufficient progesterone to maintain the lining of the uterus and for the pregnancy to implant. It is important to realize that this is not always the case. Sadly it is not uncommon to find that women who have reached their mid-thirties are producing insufficient progesterone in the second half of their cycle. This failure in progesterone levels can be enough to prevent the survival of the egg or embryo. This condition is known as luteal phase progesterone deficiency.

The cause of this failure of the corpus luteum to continue to produce quantities of progesterone is not certain. It may be a failure of the corpus luteum after ovulation and prior to fertilization, the result of which would be that the egg would not survive.

Alternatively, the failure may occur after fertilization because the embryo did not produce sufficient Human Chorionic Gonadotrophin to stimulate the corpus luteum to continue to produce progesterone. It could also be a failure of the corpus luteum to respond to the Human Chorionic Gonadotrophin.

Whatever the cause of the lack of progesterone, the effect will be the same. The endometrium will be shed and the woman will have a bleed. It can mean that either a pregnancy will never have even started or that, if it did, then an early scarriage will have occurred. Often these miscarriages are so early that they are not recognized as such and are considered to be a late period. It is helpful to know if conception has actually occurred, to help pinpoint which problems need to be addressed.

Some miscarriages that occur a little later (say at 10 or even 12 weeks) and are due to the early death of the embryo, may also be due to a lack of progesterone. However, it must be remembered that lack of progesterone is one of only several possible reasons for an early miscarriage.

Pregnancy will obviously not occur if ovulation does not take place. Anovulatory cycles – that is, cycles where the woman has a normal bleed but is not ovulating – are quite common in women, particularly from their mid-thirties onwards. Unless a woman needs to have blood tests done or some other reason to investigate her periods, this lack of ovulation can go completely unrecognized, indeed may do so for several years unless there are other symptoms. If anovulatory cycles are discovered by routine blood tests on day 20 of a 28-day cycle, then the orthodox approach is to stimulate ovulation by use of hormone treatment. This may not always be necessary, as sometimes the use of natural progesterone may stimulate the feedback mechanism between the ovary and the pituitary and re-establish the normal hormone cycle and ovulation.

Pregnancy and Birth

Once a pregnancy is established and a placenta is formed, then large amounts of progesterone – between 300 and 400 mgs per day – are produced by the placenta. This is essential to maintain the pregnancy. Once the baby has been born and the placenta, or afterbirth, has been shed, progesterone levels drop dramatically. Progesterone is one of nature's anti-depressants, and it is this sudden drop in progesterone that is responsible for the condition experienced by many women a few days after the birth of their baby – the so-called 'baby blues'. Normally this mild depression only lasts a day or two, but unfortunately with some women this depression can be prolonged and severe. This is then post-natal depression and is a very different experience to 'baby blues', so much so that some women do reject their baby during this time. Post-natal depression is very unresponsive to anti-depressants. However it frequently responds dramatically to the supplementation of natural progesterone in fairly high doses. This is logical if you consider the dramatic drop in progesterone levels that takes place at birth and the mood-elevating effects of progesterone. It is also a safe way to treat this form of depression, as natural progesterone has no side-effects and can therefore be given to a woman who is breastfeeding without any fear that it might damage her baby in any way or be passed across in the milk.

The Fertile Years – Fertility and Infertility: Questions and Answers

I AM ON THE MINI-PILL, OR PROGESTERONE-ONLY PILL, FOR CONTRACEPTION. CAN I USE NATURAL PROGESTERONE INSTEAD?
No, it would not be a good idea at all. The so-called mini-pill does not contain any progesterone at all. It contains a progestogen – a chemical that has a very powerful effect upon the lining of the uterus and cervical secretion. While the action this has is similar to that of natural progesterone, the degree of effect is very different.

While it is theoretically possible that by using natural progesterone in a high dose throughout the month you could suppress ovulation, and so prevent a pregnancy occurring, there is absolutely no guarantee that this would be the case. It depends how reliable you need your contraception to be, as this method has not been researched in terms of effectiveness. Also, you would have to use high doses of natural progesterone continuously and this would produce an abnormal hormonal state in your body, which is not desirable either.

I WOULD PREFER TO USE A NATURAL METHOD OF CONTRACEPTION RATHER THAN THE PILL. IS NATURAL PROGESTERONE A RELIABLE ALTERNATIVE?

The previous answer makes this clear, and certainly you cannot rely on progesterone to be effective in preventing a pregnancy. Progesterone is secreted naturally by the corpus luteum after ovulation. If an ovum is fertilized it secretes a hormone called Human Chorionic Gonadotrophin, which instructs the corpus luteum to carry on secreting progesterone in large quantities. This has the effect of suppressing ovulation. In theory, therefore, it should be possible to use supplements of natural progesterone to suppress ovulation and to act as a contraceptive. The drawback to this would be that it has not been researched as to reliability.

If you want to use a more natural form of contraception then you would do better to consider another method such as the Honey Cap or mucus examination, which you can be instructed in by a trained practitioner.

AFTER BEING ON THE COMBINED CONTRACEPTIVE PILL FOR MANY YEARS, I STOPPED TAKING IT SIX MONTHS AGO AND HAVE NOT HAD A PERIOD SINCE. MY DOCTOR DID A BLOOD TEST AND SAID I HAD AN EARLY MENOPAUSE AND SHOULD TAKE HRT – WHAT DO YOU THINK?

It is possible that you have had an early menopause, but if you do not have a family history of this then other explanations should be considered first. It may be that because you have been on the combined contraceptive pill for so long, the delicate feedback mechanism between the hormones of your pituitary and your ovaries has been interfered with. If this is the case, then it is possible that your pituitary hormones would be high. This happens when the pituitary is trying to stimulate the ovary to produce oestrogen. If you have reached menopause the ovary will not respond because it has reached the natural time in your life when it should stop responding. If, however, being on the Pill has made your own ovaries lazy, then they may need time to recover before they can respond.

If you supplement with natural progesterone, using it for two weeks and then stopping for two weeks, it might help to stimulate your ovaries and the feedback mechanism and your periods might well return. It is certainly worth trying this before you start on HRT. This is quite a complicated problem and you would be well advised to seek the help of a practitioner who is experienced in natural progesterone prescribing for this particular condition.

MY SEX DRIVE IS VERY LOW AND I HAVE BEEN GIVEN TESTOSTERONE BY MY DOCTOR. THIS HASN'T WORKED, AND I WONDERED IF NATURAL PROGESTERONE COULD HELP?

Some women do find that testosterone can improve their sex drive, but it by no means works in all cases. For women it is normally the rise in progesterone that occurs at the time of ovulation that is responsible for the sex drive. This is why the use of progesterone may improve libido and sex drive in some women, but it may not be the complete answer. It is important to remember that low sex drive can be due to many reasons other than a lack of hormones. Tiredness, stress, irritation with one's partner, complacency or a lack of novelty in a long-standing relationship can all be contributory factors, and you may need to address emotional as well as physical factors before seeing an improvement.

WILL NATURAL PROGESTERONE PREVENT MORNING SICKNESS IN
PREGNANCY?

There has been very little use of natural progesterone supplementation during the first few months of pregnancy – which
is when morning sickness occurs. However there is a sugges-
tion, based on a few patients' use of it, that natural progesterone may help to prevent morning sickness. You could
certainly try it as it could not do you any harm.

Also bear in mind that other alternatives have much to
offer. Herbal, homoeopathic or vitamin supplementation
can be particularly effective. Please do not attempt to dose
yourself, however, but seek out a qualified practitioner. (See
Resources page 156).

AFTER MY FIRST BABY WAS BORN I BECAME EXTREMELY DEPRESSED.
I AM NOW PREGNANT AGAIN AND DREADING ANY REOCCURRENCE,
BUT MY MIDWIFE SAID TAKING NATURAL PROGESTERONE MIGHT
HELP?

Post-natal depression is certainly due to a lack of progesterone and responds better to the use of progesterone than
anti-depressants. It is also a condition which can respond
quite dramatically in the short term.

After birth the placenta is shed and progesterone levels
in the body drop suddenly from very high to very low levels.
This is the cause of the so-called 'baby blues' that many
women experience. Normally the hormone levels balance
out and the mild depression lifts. If, however, the levels of
progesterone remain very low, the depression deepens and
carries on. This condition does not respond very well to
traditional anti-depressants, but often responds to natural
progesterone. Preferably, you should be under the direction
of a practitioner familiar with the use of natural progesterone
for this condition.

AFTER MY LAST CHILD WAS BORN I GOT THE 'BABY BLUES' QUITE
BADLY AND WAS ADVISED NOT TO BREASTFEED. WOULD NATURAL
PROGESTERONE AFFECT MY BREASTMILK?

Women are often advised to stop breastfeeding if their post-natal depression is fairly severe. The reason for this is to enable the hormone balance in the body to return to normal more quickly. If however you wish to breastfeed and are taking natural progesterone to help with the depression, then it is very unlikely to do your baby any harm even if it does enter the breastmilk. There are vast numbers of cases where mothers have continued to breastfeed one child while pregnant with the next, and they would have quite high natural levels of progesterone during the second pregnancy. No adverse effects have ever been reported from breastfeeding and taking natural progesterone at the same time.

IS IT POSSIBLE TO SUFFER FROM OESTROGEN DOMINANCE WHILE
PREGNANT OR BREASTFEEDING?

You are producing such high levels of progesterone during pregnancy that it is unlikely in the extreme that your oestrogen and progesterone levels would be out of balance, unless you are also taking oestrogen medication.

As far as breastfeeding is concerned, it is extremely unlikely that you will have high oestrogen levels – in fact oestrogen levels are often very low while breastfeeding. The reason for this is that lactation is stimulated by the pituitary hormone prolactin, and one of the other effects of this particular hormone is to reduce oestrogen levels. If you do have high oestrogen levels due to taking supplemental oestrogen during your pregnancy or after the birth, then your doctor should advise you not to breastfeed your baby. This is because there is a risk of the oestrogen being passed on through the milk. Progesterone, however, is not harmful to the baby and can safely be taken by breastfeeding mothers as a supplement if needed.

I AM IN MY LATE THIRTIES AND HAVE POSTPONED STARTING MY
FAMILY. I AM ANXIOUS TO RETAIN MY FERTILITY, AND WONDERED
IF USING NATURAL PROGESTERONE WOULD HELP ME TO DO THIS?
There is nothing to suggest that using natural progesterone
will enable you to retain your fertility any longer than nature
intended. Women's most fertile years are throughout the late
teens and twenties; we were not really designed to postpone
childbearing to a time very much later than this.

Fertility itself is a very complex subject, and the ability
to ovulate regularly and having a correct hormone balance
in the body is only one side of it. Your overall fitness, stress
levels and correct nutritional levels are also important.
Women's fertility starts to reduce naturally by the time we
have reached our mid-thirties. This seems to be due to the
fact that the monthly cycle by this age is often an anovulatory one. So your chances are reduced straight away, because
if you do not ovulate, you certainly cannot become pregnant.
Even if you do ovulate, another potential problem is that as
you become older it seems that the ovary does not always
produce enough progesterone to enable the egg and embryo
to survive. If a lack of progesterone is shown to be a problem
when you reach the point of trying for a pregnancy, then
supplementation with natural progesterone might help; certainly it would be sensible to consult with fertility special-
ists in the field of nutritional supplementation, who can be
extremely helpful. You will find some therapists listed in the
Resources chapter.

MY PARTNER AND I HAVE BEEN TRYING TO BECOME PREGNANT
BUT WITHOUT SUCCESS. WHAT COULD BE GOING WRONG?
Becoming pregnant is not as easy as we imagine. Even when
there are no problems at all there are only two or at most
three days each month when pregnancy can occur, and even
this does not happen every month, as occasionally the fallopian tubes fail to catch the egg!

In the second half of the menstrual cycle, after ovulation, the hormone progesterone should be secreted by the ovary in large quantities. Its functions are to maintain the viability of the egg so that it can be fertilized and to maintain the lining of the uterus in a condition that will allow a fertilized egg to implant and develop. If for some reason there is a lack of progesterone in the second half of the menstrual cycle, there may be difficulty in fertilizing an egg. Or if the egg becomes fertilized and sufficient progesterone does not continue to be made by the ovary until the placenta forms, then early miscarriage may occur. In these cases the use of progesterone in the second half of the menstrual cycle and during the first three months of pregnancy is helpful.

It can seem like an agonizingly long time when you are trying to become pregnant, and your state of mind is an important factor. Consulting someone who has experience of using natural progesterone to help fertility would be a good step; you will find some therapists listed in the Resources chapter.

I AM IN MY MID-FORTIES AND HAVE STARTED A NEW RELATIONSHIP. WE WOULD LIKE TO HAVE A BABY BUT WONDER IF IT'S TOO DIFFICULT AT MY AGE.

There are a number of reasons why it is more difficult to become pregnant when you are in your forties. One of these reasons can be that, even if you are ovulating, your ovaries may not be making the normal amount of progesterone in the second half of your cycle. If you do not make enough progesterone after you have ovulated the egg will not survive long enough to be fertilized, or even if it does become fertilized the embryo may not survive. Yet another problem which can arise is that if the level of progesterone drops, the lining of the uterus will be shed and the embryo will not be able to implant and will be washed away with the menstrual flow.

Supplementing with natural progesterone could well help, and could certainly not do any harm. It would be useful to have the guidance of a practitioner experienced in the use of natural progesterone for this purpose, as adjusting the dosage is critical. The natural progesterone should be used in the second half of the cycle after ovulation; if you suspect that a pregnancy has occurred, the progesterone should not be stopped until the third month of pregnancy. By this time the placenta will be making enough progesterone to support the baby.

I am sure that you will investigate all possibilities, but do not forget that your partner will also need to undergo a series of tests as well.

I HAVE A FAMILY HISTORY OF OSTEOPOROSIS AND AM TAKING NATURAL PROGESTERONE TO MAINTAIN MY BONES. I WISH TO START A FAMILY NEXT YEAR, SO DO I KEEP ON TAKING THE NATURAL PROGESTERONE DURING THAT TIME?

This is a tricky one to answer, as taking natural progesterone for osteoporosis is a long-term treatment. Generally speaking, if you are using natural progesterone and trying to become pregnant it is essential that you have the advice of an experienced practitioner before you start planning your family. This is because it is critical that you do not interfere with ovulation; it can be a delicate task to get the balance right.

NATURAL PROGESTERONE IS A GODSEND FOR MY PMS, BUT I AM ALSO TRYING TO GET PREGNANT. WILL IT STOP ME DOING THAT?

You are probably in fact improving your chance of a pregnancy by using it. Progesterone is the hormone secreted in large quantities by a woman when she is pregnant. During pregnancy the placenta produces in the region of 400 mg of progesterone per day. If you are supplementing with one of the progesterone creams you will be getting only a fraction of that, around 20 to 30 mg per day.

During a normal menstrual cycle the ovary produces progesterone following ovulation – that is, in the second half of your cycle, from about day 14 until menstruation. If you are using natural progesterone for PMS you should be using it in the second half of your cycle, that is to say during the part of your cycle when your own body will normally produce it. The fact that you have PMS indicates that you do not usually produce enough natural progesterone yourself during that time. If you are trying to become pregnant you should take great care each month not to stop using the natural progesterone, even if you think you may be pregnant. If enough progesterone is not produced after ovulation, a fertilized egg cannot survive and your body cannot sustain the new life.

I HAVE HAD PROBLEMS IN THE PAST WITH MISCARRIAGES. I AM USING NATURAL PROGESTERONE, BUT SHOULD I CONTINUE WITH IT WHEN I AM NEXT PREGNANT?

There is no reason for you to stop using natural progesterone when you become pregnant, and certainly if you have been using it to prevent an early miscarriage then it is vital that you do not stop taking it when you become pregnant again. Normally as soon as an egg is fertilized it starts to secrete the hormone Human Chorionic Gonadotrophin. This hormone stimulates the corpus luteum (in the ovary from which the egg ovulated) to secrete lots of progesterone. This should continue until the placenta forms and produces large amounts of progesterone to support the baby. Sometimes, though, the corpus luteum does not respond as well as it should to the Human Chorionic Gonadotrophin and doesn't secrete much progesterone. If this happens, then the endometrial lining of the uterus may be shed and an early miscarriage will result. This is why if you are using natural progesterone to prevent an early miscarriage you must continue to use even larger amounts of natural progesterone when you become pregnant, until your own body's production takes over.

I HAVE BEEN HAVING VARIOUS FORMS OF IVF TREATMENT.
FOLLOWING IMPLANTATION OF THE FERTILIZED EGGS, I HAVE
BEEN GIVEN CYCLOGEST (A PROGESTERONE SUPPOSITORY) TO USE
FOR ABOUT TWO WEEKS. EVERYTHING HAS GONE WELL UNTIL I
STOP THE CYCLOGEST. THEN I MISCARRY. I THINK USING NATURAL
PROGESTERONE MIGHT HELP, BUT MY CONSULTANT SAYS NOT.

Each Cyclogest suppository delivers quite a high dosage – either 200 mg or 400 mg of natural progesterone. The Cyclogest is given to ensure that there is a normal, or near normal, hormonal balance in your body following the insertion of the fertilized egg. The reasoning behind the fairly short-term use of the Cyclogest is that the embryo will implant rapidly in the uterus and the placenta will then produce enough progesterone to keep the pregnancy going. While this is often the case, it appears that sometimes it takes longer for the embryo to implant and longer for the placenta to get going than is often realized. You could discuss this with your consultant and say that you would like to see the effect of using the Cyclogest for a much longer period to see what happens. The important thing is that using Cyclogest for this relatively short period of time will not produce any side-effects or cause any damage to the foetus, and it just might work.

You would need to use Cyclogest or Crinone gel in order to maintain the initial high levels of progesterone. The various creams available would probably not be strong enough.

I HAVE BEEN TAKING NATURAL PROGESTERONE AND AM NOW
PREGNANT. SHOULD I CONTINUE WITH IT THROUGHOUT MY
PREGNANCY?

During pregnancy progesterone is vital, as without it no baby could ever survive and be born. However, the body is very efficient and once the placenta has been formed it makes large amounts of progesterone, up to 400 mg per day. In fact the placenta forms quite early in pregnancy, and is producing increasing quantities of progesterone by the eighth week. In these circumstances you can see that there is no need for you to continue taking the progesterone, unless you were originally taking it for luteal phase progesterone deficiency. If that is the case, then follow the directions in the next question.

I HAVE BEEN TAKING NATURAL PROGESTERONE FOR LUTEAL PHASE
INFERTILITY. DO I STOP TAKING IT WHEN I BECOME PREGNANT?
Progesterone is essential to ensure that an early pregnancy is not miscarried. If you have had a luteal phase deficiency of progesterone this is because your corpus luteum after ovulation has not been able to make enough progesterone. During the first few weeks of pregnancy, before the placenta is formed, the ability of the foetus to survive is dependent on progesterone from the corpus luteum. As your corpus luteum has not been doing this very well on its own, it is very important to continue with your supplementation of natural progesterone until about week 10 or 12 of your pregnancy. If you stop supplementation as soon as you discover that you are pregnant you will cause a sudden drop in progesterone levels. This could cause the lining of the uterus to be shed, which will result in an early miscarriage.

WOMEN OFTEN GET VARICOSE VEINS DURING PREGNANCY, AND I
AM CONCERNED BECAUSE I AM TAKING NATURAL PROGESTERONE
AT THE MOMENT. WILL TAKING NATURAL PROGESTERONE MAKE IT
MORE LIKELY I WILL GET VARICOSE VEINS WHEN I AM PREGNANT?
The cause of varicose veins during pregnancy is not related to high progesterone levels. It is due to the weight of the baby in the uterus pressing on the veins in the abdomen. The pressure on these veins obstructs the flow of blood from the veins in the legs, so that they tend to become varicosed.

CHAPTER 4

Menopause

Often it can be quite confusing for a woman to know when her menopause is really occurring. There are many symptoms and changes that arise in the time before menopause proper, when the periods stop altogether. This time is known as pre-menopause, and although the majority of women experience it for varying lengths of time, there are some for whom the pre-menopause simply never happens. They suddenly realize that they have not had a period for several months, have had no other symptoms, and have reached their menopause. These are the lucky ones. Because symptoms flow across this whole time period, pre-menopause and menopause are discussed here together, to help women identify common problems that can occur during both phases.

PRE-MENOPAUSE – INTRODUCTION

Unfortunately, for many women the pre-menopause can be a time of various problems. These nearly all arise because of the changes that are taking place in the hormone balance of the body. As with menopause itself, the age at which the pre-menopause begins can vary from woman to woman. It may start as early as the late thirties or as late as the late forties. It is often characterized by irregular menstruation. This is usually due to the fact that ovulation is not occurring on a regular basis, and as a result the hormone balance is disturbed. When ovulation does not occur and the oestrogen levels are still high in relation to progesterone, as they will be during menopause, symptoms of oestrogen dominance are apparent. You will find the list of oestrogen-dominance symptoms on page 5,6 and 39.

If there is no ovulation, then no progesterone is formed by the ovary to balance the oestrogen levels. Even if ovulation does occur, there can still be a failure by the ovary to make enough progesterone to balance the oestrogen. This is known as luteal phase progesterone deficiency, and again symptoms of oestrogen dominance will occur. Even if the periods are still regular, a woman can still not be ovulating, and so not producing progesterone. Women who are looking to start their families in their late thirties and early forties will find that their doctor will look first at whether they are having anovulatory cycles, as these are an obvious cause of infertility in women at this time in life.

Most women who are experiencing a difficult transition through their pre-menopausal years will find their symptoms eased by natural progesterone supplementation, as it will help balance the oestrogen which is still being produced in large amounts.

Pre-Menopause: Questions and Answers

AFTER YEARS ON A COMBINED CONTRACEPTIVE PILL, I CAME OFF SIX MONTHS AGO AND HAVEN'T HAD A PERIOD SINCE. MY DOCTOR SAYS I'M HAVING AN EARLY MENOPAUSE, BUT I AM ONLY 37. SURELY THIS IS TOO YOUNG?

It is possible that you have had an early menopause, but if you do not have a family history of this then other explanations should be considered first. Such a long time on a combined

Pill could have affected the delicate feedback mechanism between the hormones of your pituitary and your ovaries. If this is the case, then it is possible that your pituitary hormones would be high. This happens when the pituitary is trying to stimulate the ovary to produce oestrogen. If you have genuinely reached menopause, the ovary will not respond because it has reached the natural time in your life when it should stop responding. If, however, being on the Pill has made your own ovaries lazy, then they may need time to recover before they can respond.

If you supplement with natural progesterone, using it for two weeks and then stopping for two weeks, it might help to stimulate your ovaries and the feedback mechanism and your periods might well return. It is certainly worth trying this before you start on HRT. This is quite a complicated problem and you would be well advised to seek the help of a practitioner who is experienced in natural progesterone prescribing for this particular condition.

I AM IN MY EARLY FORTIES AND MY PERIODS HAVE BECOME VERY IRREGULAR. COULD NATURAL PROGESTERONE HELP?

In the mid-thirties and early forties it is not uncommon for women to stop ovulating. When that happens, because you are still pre-menopausal your ovaries will continue to make large amounts of oestrogen. This builds up the endometrium, or lining of the uterus. When the lining becomes very thick it will tend to shed itself and you will bleed.

Because you are not ovulating, you will not be making very much progesterone so there will be no control over the bleeding and it will occur in an erratic way. If you supplement with natural progesterone the aim will be to use it during the two weeks you would expect to be the second half of your menstrual cycle – that is from day 14 to 28 if you are on a 28-day cycle. If your periods are very erratic and have been for some time, then it can take several cycles before you begin to see a return to regularity.

I AM HAVING HEAVY, PROLONGED BLEEDING EACH MONTH. I HAVE
BEEN TOLD THIS IS BECAUSE I AM PRE-MENOPAUSAL. MY DOCTOR
HAS PRESCRIBED NORETHISTERONE, WHICH MAKES ME FEEL ILL.
WOULD NATURAL PROGESTERONE BE BETTER FOR ME?

Your heavy, prolonged bleeding is probably due to the fact
that you have stopped ovulating. When you stop ovulating
the ovaries do not produce progesterone and the bleeding
tends to become prolonged. It is sometimes possible to control this heavy, prolonged bleeding with natural progesterone, but it is not easy. You will need the help of a medical
practitioner because you may still need to use some norethisterone at times when the natural progesterone is just not
strong enough to control the bleeding. It can take several
months to control the bleeding this way, but is well worth
trying. It is also important to correct any anaemia which
might have resulted from your prolonged heavy bleeding.
See the question on depression and tiredness on pages 80 and
104 for suggestions on dealing with anaemia.

I AM IN MY EARLY FORTIES. MY PERIODS ARE VERY REGULAR BUT I
HAVE STARTED TO HAVE PMS FOR A WEEK BEFORE MY PERIOD. I
HAVE NEVER HAD THIS BEFORE. WOULD NATURAL PROGESTERONE
HELP ME?

The onset of PMS during the pre-menopausal years is yet
another example of what happens when we start to have
anovulatory cycles. Although you are having regular periods
you are probably not ovulating, or if you are ovulating your
ovaries are not making the normal amount of progesterone
in the second half of your cycle. As a result you are oestrogen-dominant, which means the amount of oestrogen you
are making is not being balanced by enough progesterone.

When you have oestrogen dominance you will develop
some or all of associated symptoms associated with unopposed oestrogen. If you read through the list that appears on
page 39, you will recognize many of the effects as being what

we know as PMS. These include bloating, painful breasts, irritability and mood swings.

This situation can certainly be helped by supplementing with natural progesterone. The best way would be to use it during the second half of your cycle.

MY ALTERNATIVE PRACTITIONER HAS TOLD ME THAT THE
SYMPTOMS I HAVE SUGGEST OESTROGEN DOMINANCE. I AM
NEARING MY MENOPAUSE AND MY DOCTOR HAS TOLD ME THAT MY
OESTROGEN LEVELS ARE FALLING. HOW CAN I BE OESTROGEN
DOMINANT?

When we speak of oestrogen dominance we are referring to the ratio of oestrogen to progesterone and the fact that these two hormones need to be balanced. No one has yet worked out what, or indeed if, there is an exact ratio which can be measured. It probably cannot.

The way in which oestrogen dominance is recognized is by the symptoms which the woman presents. If you consult the list of oestrogen and progesterone effects on page 4, you will see that most of them counter-balance each other. If progesterone is lacking then the effects of the oestrogen are the most pronounced and oestrogen dominance exists. This imbalance can occur both at high levels of oestrogen and at low levels of oestrogen. Your practitioner is probably correct in her diagnosis because you are pre-menopausal, and at this time the ovaries often stop producing sufficient amounts of progesterone to balance your oestrogens.

MY DOCTOR HAS TOLD ME THAT BECAUSE I AM NEARING
MENOPAUSE I SHOULD TAKE HRT TO PROTECT MYSELF FROM HEART
DISEASE AND OSTEOPOROSIS. I FEEL PERFECTLY WELL, SO WHY DO I
NEED TO TAKE IT?

If you are feeling perfectly well, even though you are approaching menopause there is absolutely no reason at all to start taking either HRT or indeed any natural progesterone.

Traditional HRT and natural progesterone are both hormones and should only be taken if and when you have symptoms which suggest that you need them. Please do remember that menopause is a natural passage of life, and that there is no reason at all why you should automatically suffer health problems.

There is a great deal of nonsense spoken about menopause – often by people who should know better. HRT will not protect you from either osteoporosis or heart disease, and provides no guarantee of a trouble-free menopause. Indeed many women find the associated side-effects of HRT more distressing than menopausal symptoms themselves.

MY DOCTOR WANTS ME TO TAKE HRT EVEN THOUGH I AM ONLY 42.
I THINK I AM PRE-MENOPAUSAL, AND AM CONCERNED ABOUT
OSTEOPOROSIS.

In spite of what some doctors will tell you, not everyone develops osteoporosis. One sensible precaution if you are concerned is to ask your doctor to arrange for you to have a bone density scan. Osteoporosis cannot be diagnosed any other way, and certainly not by looking at you or estimating your risk because of family or your own medical history. With a scan, if there is a problem you will be able to diagnose it in the very early stages. If the scan shows that you have a lowered density then definitely you would benefit from making sure you have a good diet, do weight-bearing exercises, take specific supplements such as calcium, magnesium and boron, and make sure you get adequate supplementation with natural progesterone to build up new bone. HRT will not build up new bone, only slow down the rate at which you lose old bone. You want to be looking forward to many years of building up strong, constantly renewing bone – and only natural progesterone, not HRT, can do this.

MY NEW PARTNER WANTS US TO HAVE A BABY, BUT I AM PRE-
MENOPAUSAL. HAVE WE LEFT IT TOO LATE?

It may not be too late, but it is not going to be as easy and
straightforward as when you were younger. You are probably
not ovulating regularly, and unlikely to be making sufficient
progesterone in the second half of your cycle. It's essential to
have sufficient progesterone for the egg to survive long
enough to be fertilized, and then to have enough progesterone to support a viable foetus.

Your best plan would be to talk to a specialist who works
with natural progesterone and fertility, as adjusting the
dosage is fairly skilled. Normally you would supplement
with natural progesterone in the second half of your cycle
after ovulation. If you have reason then to think that a pregnancy has occurred, do not stop using natural progesterone
until at least the third month of your pregnancy. By this time
the placenta will be making enough of its own progesterone.

I AM PRE-MENOPAUSAL AND AM FINDING IT VERY DIFFICULT TO
CONTROL MY WEIGHT. I DIET AND TAKE EXERCISE, BUT CANNOT
SHIFT IT. THIS NEVER USED TO BE A PROBLEM FOR ME WHEN I WAS
YOUNGER, AND I WONDER IF NATURAL PROGESTERONE WOULD
HELP?

It is most likely that you are no longer making sufficient
progesterone to balance your oestrogen. One of the effects of
oestrogen is to build up fat, and one of the effects of progesterone is to enable the body to break down excess fat.
Oestrogen also retains fluid, whereas progesterone helps the
body eliminate it. For many women around pre-menopausal
time, fluid retention is an important factor that adds to their
weight problem. Many of these symptoms relate to oestrogen
dominance, so supplementing with natural progesterone
could well make it easier for you to control your weight.

I AM PRE-MENOPAUSAL AND FOR NO REASON THAT I CAN THINK OF HAVE STARTED TO FEEL VERY DEPRESSED. MY DOCTOR HAS SUGGESTED PROZAC, BUT WOULD NATURAL PROGESTERONE DO ANYTHING FOR THIS?

Progesterone is the body's own natural anti-depressant. Because you are approaching menopause your ovaries are probably not making enough progesterone to balance your oestrogen. Oestrogen can make you feel depressed if it is not balanced by sufficient progesterone. Try natural progesterone first, and also perhaps consult with an alternative practitioner such as a homoeopath or herbalist. Many women find a supplement containing hypericum (also known as St John's Wort), Kava Kava or Schizandra very effective at helping with depression at this time of life.

I HAVE HAD FIBROIDS FOR MANY YEARS, AND NOW MY DOCTOR WANTS ME TO TAKE HRT BECAUSE I AM PRE-MENOPAUSAL. I AM WORRIED ABOUT THIS AS I BELIEVE IT COULD MAKE MY FIBROIDS WORSE?

If you are not experiencing any symptoms then there is no need for you to start HRT. Menopause is not a disease and we do not need to take HRT just because we are approaching it.

If you are suffering with severe symptoms, then HRT might be useful. But if your fibroids are not causing you any discomfort then they are no reason to put you on HRT. In fact for you to takc HRT would be unwise, because the large amounts of oestrogen contained in it would feed your fibroids and they could grow rapidly. Because of this the often-suggested next step is that you have a hysterectomy; sadly much surgery performed in this way may be totally unnecessary.

If you have no symptoms or problems from your fibroids then leave well enough alone. When you reach your menopause the fibroids will naturally begin to shrink. If your fibroids are causing you some problems or they seem to be

growing, then certainly supplementing with natural progesterone could be useful. Natural progesterone rarely reduces
the size of fibroids, but it can sometimes stop them from
becoming any larger. You may also find it helpful to read the
questions on fibroids in Chapter 3.

I AM IN MY LATE FORTIES AND PRESUME THAT I AM PRE-
MENOPAUSAL ALTHOUGH THERE HAS BEEN NO CHANGE IN MY
MONTHLY CYCLE. THE ONE THING THAT HAS STARTED TO BOTHER
ME IS THAT MY BREASTS HAVE BECOME VERY LUMPY AND TENDER.
Tender and lumpy breasts are a classic symptom of oestrogen
dominance. This is a common situation in the pre-menopausal
years and is due to the fact that although the ovary still
makes plenty of oestrogen, either ovulation does not occur
or, if it does, the ovary does not make the normal amount of
progesterone needed. If you have oestrogen dominance then
the natural stimulating effect of oestrogen on breast tissue
will not be balanced by progesterone. The breast tissue then
becomes over-stimulated, and cysts can form.

Another problem can be that fluid retention occurs in the
breasts and this can make them swell and be very tender.
Supplementation with natural progesterone for three weeks
out of four in your cycle could help to restore the oestrogen-
to-progesterone balance and solve the problem with your
breasts. You should be warned that sometimes the breast
tenderness becomes worse when you start using the progesterone before it gets better.

I AM PRE-MENOPAUSAL. I FEEL WELL AND HAVE NO SYMPTOMS
WHICH I CAN RELATE TO HORMONE IMBALANCE, BUT I AM VERY
TIRED AND DO NOT HAVE AS MUCH ENERGY AS I USED TO.
While it is unpleasant to be reminded of the fact, we should
not expect to have quite as much energy in our forties as we
did in our twenties. Also we women tend to lead very stressful and busy lives today. It's important to remember the time

of approaching menopause is intended by nature to be one during which a woman should step back a bit and review her life and how she spends her time.

Many hormonal and other changes are naturally taking place, and these processes in the body do use up energy. Natural progesterone will only help your tiredness if it is related to oestrogen dominance. It is worth trying it to see if it has the effect of lifting your energy, but you should look at other factors in your life, too.

I AM IN MY MID-FORTIES AND HAVE ALWAYS TAKEN CARE OF MYSELF AND DONE EVERYTHING POSSIBLE TO KEEP MYSELF LOOKING YOUNG. I DREAD THE MENTAL AND PHYSICAL DETERIORATION OF MENOPAUSE. I AM ATTRACTED TO TAKING HRT SO AS TO KEEP MY LOOKS, BUT AM CONCERNED BECAUSE OF A STRONG FAMILY HISTORY OF BREAST CANCER.

The most important thing for you to realize is that reaching menopause does *not* mean mental and physical deterioration. Nor does it mean you suddenly become old. Menopause is natural, and while admittedly old age cannot be put off for ever it does not suddenly descend upon us at menopause. If you have always looked after your body and your health then that is a wonderful foundation for a healthy later life, but it is just as important to have a positive attitude to menopause. Certainly if you have a strong family history of breast cancer you should avoid HRT because the risk of breast cancer for you would be a high one. It is also unlikely that any doctor would prescribe HRT for someone with your family history.

Many of the promises made with regard to HRT and how it will keep you forever young have absolutely no proven basis. They are an attractive sales pitch to woo women to take a drug that on the whole many reject because of side-effects and known health risks.

In order to protect your breasts you would be well advised to consider taking natural progesterone to counteract the effects of oestrogen dominance as you enter menopause. Do remember, though, that neither HRT nor natural progesterone is an elixir of youth.

You might also find it helpful to read the section on cancer and natural progesterone on page 109.

I AM PRE-MENOPAUSAL. IF I START USING NATURAL PROGESTERONE NOW WILL IT POSTPONE MENOPAUSE?
We do not know what makes menopause happen when it does. If we did, we might be able to postpone it. Women have used natural progesterone now for many years, and although it helps make the transition through menopause easier and healthier, there is nothing to suggest that using natural progesterone postpones its onset.

I AM IN MY EARLY FORTIES AND MY HAIR HAS BECOME DRY AND LIFELESS. IS THIS HORMONAL?
It is possible that natural progesterone could help you to improve the quality of your hair, as hormone imbalance does affect it. Certainly many women notice a distinct change in the texture of their hair around this time. When a woman is pregnant she often has very lovely hair, and that is a time when her progesterone levels are very high. You could supplement with natural progesterone and see what happens, but do not expect a result too quickly. Hair which has been damaged takes months to fall out, and months to grow again.

MENOPAUSE – INTRODUCTION

Strictly speaking, menopause actually means last period. In common use, however, the term 'menopause' has come to cover a much longer period of time. Women who are either pre- or post-menopausal often find themselves included within this group, as some symptoms seem to occur across all these categories. So when we use the word menopause here, it can also include all women from their early forties, or even late thirties, onwards.

When a woman's periods cease finally, then that is the end of her reproductive life. What it most definitely does *not* mean is the end of a woman's useful life. Menopause is a time that is often anticipated with gloom and despair. This is not a healthy attitude, and women who approach their menopause in this spirit are often setting themselves up to have the very problems they are dreading.

It is true that many women do experience some difficulties at this time of life, but the important thing to remember is that most of these can be dealt with quite straightforwardly.

Menopause occurs in women for a very good biological reason. It is not a curse wrought on us at a time in our lives when we are looking forward to enjoying active, healthy and childcare-free years. If there were no cessation of fertility, as occurs at menopause, how many of us would want to continue having babies or having to take precautions against pregnancy all our lives? Also, in evolutionary terms babies need to have parents young and healthy enough to be around long enough to rear them into adulthood. If we continued to be pregnant into our sixties, seventies and eighties, who would bring up our children? As a species we would soon be extinct if we could not fulfil this most primary of parental tasks, that of living long enough to see our children established as young adults.

It is often stated today by 'experts' that the problems of menopause did not occur commonly in past generations because women did not live long enough to reach this landmark. To support this theory, they tell us that the life expectancy of women a generation or so ago was only about 45, whereas now it is 75. This is true – and is a damning example of how statistics will mislead you. Life expectancy is based on an average of the length of life – logical enough. Women a generation or so ago had the statistics massively stacked against them because of two factors. First, many babies died before their first birthday, and secondly, many women died in childbirth. This resulted in a considerable number of women having only very short lives. However, those women who survived these two major hazards often lived as long or longer than we can expect to now. You only have to walk round a cemetery and look at the gravestones to confirm this. You will find many women buried there who lived to a very good age, and we know that women over the age of 50 will have experienced menopause, so to say it is a modern phenomenon because women are now living longer is simply not true.

The Pattern of Menopause

We do not know what causes menopause to happen any more than we know what triggers puberty. It may be a built-in age-ing process either in the pituitary mechanism or in the ovary itself. It used to be suggested that it was because the ovary ran out of eggs. This does not seem to be the case, as recent events have shown that elderly women well after their nat-ural menopause can with the supplementary use of strong hormones be made to ovulate and even produce eggs which can be fertilized.

What does happen is that the hormone balance changes, and that anovulatory cycles (where no ovulation happens) may occur. The menstrual cycle also tends to become more irregular, and higher levels of pituitary hormones are pro-duced in an attempt to stimulate the ovaries. After a few months or years the hormone balance settles down to a new pattern. The Follicular Stimulating Hormone (FSH) levels of the pituitary often remain high, but the ovary no longer responds to it. As a result of this lack of response, the levels of the oestrogens in the body also drop. In fact the balance of the oestrogens themselves changes. Instead of our main oestrogen being oestradiol (which is produced mainly in the ovary), the dominant oestrogen becomes oestrone. This particular oestrogen is made in the fatty tissue of the body from androstenedione, which is made in the adrenals. Levels of progesterone, which is the other ovarian hormone, drop dramatically because we no longer ovulate and do not therefore have any corpus luteum from which to make this hormone. It continues to be made by the adrenals, but in much smaller quantities.

It is this new hormone balance which is the key to how we feel during menopause. If our oestrogens and progesterone remain balanced then we feel well. If they do not, as is the case for a substantial number of women, then we do not feel well. The problems of menopause are so often stated as being due to a lack of oestrogen, but this is often not the case. It is far more usual for the problems to be due to a lack of progesterone, or as it has been referred to, 'oestrogen dominance'. This is a difficult idea for many people – including doctors – to grasp because we know that oestrogens drop at menopause, so how can they be dominant? They can because it is the *ratio* of oestrogen to progesterone that matters. The effect of this imbalance is the same whether the levels are high or low. If the ratio is wrong, then there can be oestrogen dominance. It is perhaps easier to understand if we think of it not so much as oestrogen dominance as a lack of progesterone.

A commonly asked question is why does this happen? If menopause is natural and should happen easily in all women, then what has gone wrong? Has mother nature made a mistake? No, mother nature has not made any mistakes – we have. As a result of our lifestyles, diet, pollution, stress, drugs and environmental pollutants we have created a situation where oestrogens abound in far greater quantities than could ever have been envisaged. Hot flushes (or flashes as they are known in the USA), night sweats, dry vagina, mood swings, osteoporosis – all these are being experienced by many women at menopause, and are a direct result of this imbalance between progesterone and oestrogen.

On pages 4–5 you will find two lists to refer to: one of these gives the effects of oestrogens and the other the effects of progesterone on the body. You will recognize many given on the list of oestrogen effects as the symptoms of menopausal problems. This shows that they are due to unopposed oestrogen, and explains why these symptoms generally respond well to supplementation with natural progesterone.

Menopause: Questions and Answers

HOW DO I COME OFF HRT AND REPLACE IT WITH PROGESTERONE?
Slowly. Take two to three months to gradually cut down the amount of oestrogen you are taking. Although some women do stop HRT suddenly and feel no ill-effects it is better to do this over a period of time to allow your body to adjust.

It is essential that you stop taking the synthetic progestagen part of your HRT immediately you begin supplementing with natural progesterone. <u>You cannot take the two together</u>, so you need to ensure you are on a form of HRT that is oestrogen-only. Ask your doctor to switch you if you are on a combined pill or patch, and tell him or her you wish to substitute the natural progesterone for the progestogen part of the regime.

During the first month you want to cut your oestrogen intake by a quarter. If you are free of oestrogen dominance symptoms on this dose, then in the second month cut down to a half and in the third month cut down to a quarter. By the fourth month, if you are symptom-free, you should be able to stop the oestrogen altogether. You will need to monitor your progress. It is advisable to go slowly and you can stay at the same oestrogen dosage for several months if that is helping your symptoms. The aim is to cut down gradually.

HOW DO I REDUCE MY OESTROGEN INTAKE WHEN MY DOCTOR SAYS MY BRAND OF HRT IS A LOW DOSE ANYWAY?

The instructions are the same for most brands of HRT, but if you are on a high dose of oestrogen then the advice in the following question will be more applicable to you. For most women their HRT will be in the form of patches or pills, and the following is a tried and trusted method of coming off.

If you are on oestrogen patches, then begin the first month of supplementation with progesterone by reducing the size of the patch by a quarter. Just cut it with scissors, or put an adhesive band or sticking plaster with a hole cut out of the centre on top of the patch, adhesive to adhesive. This will reduce the amount of oestrogen in contact with your skin.

If you are on a Pill, cut it so you are only taking three-quarters of it during the first month, then half the second month, a quarter in the third and stop altogether in the fourth month. Please remember that you must monitor your symptoms and adjust the oestrogen to be at the level where you are comfortable and symptom-free. If in doubt, consult with a doctor who is experienced in the prescribing of natural progesterone. You can obtain a list of these from the Natural Progesterone Information Service (see the Resources chapter).

I WANT TO COME OFF HRT. I HAVE BEEN TOLD THAT I MUST STOP TAKING THE PROGESTOGEN PART OF MY HRT AND REPLACE IT WITH NATURAL PROGESTERONE. WILL MY UTERUS BE PROTECTED WHILE I DO THIS?

If you are able to make this change from HRT to natural progesterone over three months then you do not need to worry about your endometrium not being protected, as hyperplasia (over-stimulation of the uterus, which can lead to the development of pre-cancerous cells) is unlikely to occur in such a short time. Certainly the oestrogen will continue to have an effect on the lining of the uterus, but as you rapidly reduce the levels of oestrogen the natural progesterone cream should be sufficient to protect it and prevent the lining being built up.

If your particular brand of HRT contains a high dose of oestrogen, or you find that you cannot reduce the oestrogen levels quickly enough, then you should not rely on natural progesterone cream to protect the endometrium. The best way to come off your HRT in these circumstances is to change the progestogen part of your HRT for progesterone tablets or pessaries which are of a higher dose than the cream. At the same time you should gradually reduce your level of oestrogen until you experience little or no bleeding following the use of the progesterone tablets or pessaries. Then it is safe to change over to the natural progesterone cream and either maintain that level of oestrogen if you need it, or continue to slowly reduce the amount of oestrogen you are taking.

I HAVE RECENTLY CHANGED FROM MY TRADITIONAL HRT TO TAKING OESTROGEN AND NATURAL PROGESTERONE. I TAKE THE OESTROGEN EVERY DAY AND THE NATURAL PROGESTERONE TOGETHER WITH THE OESTROGEN FOR 10 DAYS EACH MONTH. WHEN I WAS ON HRT I HAD A BLEED EVERY MONTH, BUT THIS HAS NOT HAPPENED SINCE I CHANGED OVER AND I AM WORRIED THAT MY UTERUS MAY NOT BE PROTECTED.

You are right to be concerned that your uterus may not be being protected. You must discuss this with your doctor. What may be happening is that the progesterone dosage needs to be adjusted to ensure a bleed. If your doctor feels that your dosages are balanced and that you do not need to bleed because the endometrium is not building up, then you have no cause to worry. If your doctor is not sure whether the dosage is correct or not, then an ultrasound scan of your uterus will soon tell whether or not the endometrium is building up.

I AM TAKING HRT. I FEEL FINE WHEN I AM JUST TAKING THE OESTROGEN. I BEGIN TO FEEL UNWELL AS SOON AS I START TAKING THE PROGESTOGEN. CAN I REPLACE THE PROGESTOGEN WITH PROGESTERONE?

There is no reason at all why you should not replace the progestogen with natural progesterone. The important thing is to ensure that you take a sufficient dosage of natural progesterone to protect the endometrium. Oestrogen has the effect of building up the lining of the uterus, and if this is not prevented from happening, or if it does happen and is not shed as a bleed each month, then hyperplasia – which can lead to cancer – could occur. If you take natural progesterone for 10 days each month, and if the oestrogen has built up the endometrium, then a bleed will occur.

ON HRT I HAD A BLEED REGULARLY EVERY MONTH. SINCE I STARTED TAKING NATURAL PROGESTERONE I HAVE NOT HAD A PERIOD AT ALL. IS THIS USUAL?

There can be a period of adjustment, and for some women the HRT causes a bleed to happen when the body may not have continued to do so on its own, so when you stop, the artificially-induced bleeding will also stop. Having said this, there are other factors to consider as well. Ask your doctor to arrange for an ultrasound scan of your uterus so that you can tell whether or not the endometrium is building up. If it isn't, then there is no need to worry because no bleeding should be happening. If it is building up, however, then it must be dispersed, and it may be that the progesterone dosage needs to be adjusted to ensure a bleed.

I AM TAKING HRT. IF I START TAKING PROGESTERONE WILL I GET
A BLEED?

It depends on whether you are actually through the
menopause and have reached the end of your cycle or if you
have not been bleeding because of some other hormone-
related factor. If the lining of your womb is still being built
up by oestrogen, and you are also taking natural progesterone
for 10 days each month, then a bleed will normally occur. If
you are truly through menopause and no womb lining is
being built up, then progesterone will not bring on a bleed, as
there will be nothing there to be expelled.

CAN YOU USE NATURAL PROGESTERONE AND OESTROGENS
TOGETHER?

Progesterone and oestrogens occur naturally together in the
body in balance, so there is no reason why you should not use
them together if your symptoms indicate that you need to.
Oestrogens are frequently used on their own by women
who have had hysterectomies with or without the removal of
their ovaries. This is not good for the body, as it produces a
severe imbalance; the oestrogens should be combined with
natural progesterone. You will probably need the help of your
practitioner to decide what combination is correct for you.

I WANT TO SWITCH MY HRT TO USING NATURAL PROGESTERONE
AND OESTROGEN, BUT MY GYNAECOLOGIST HAS TOLD ME IT WILL
INCREASE MY RISK OF ENDOMETRIAL CANCER. IS HE RIGHT?

Using a combination of oestrogen and progesterone cream
will definitely *not* increase the risk of endometrial cancer.
Long-term use of oestrogen on its own will increase your risk
of endometrial cancer, but if you are intending to supplement with natural progesterone then this risk will be considerably reduced.

HRT in its early days consisted of just oestrogen, and
endometrial cancer was a risk for women taking no

progesterone supplementation. What happened was that in order to protect the uterus from the oestrogen, the drug companies added in a synthetic form of progesterone, a progestogen, to make sure a woman got a monthly bleed to get rid of the lining of the womb which had built up and prevent it becoming cancerous. However, if you are on a traditional form of HRT which has high dosages of oestrogen, you can still get an increase in the lining of the uterus, even when progestogens are used.

While it has been shown that natural progesterone can protect the endometrium against the stimulating effects of extra oestrogen, if you are on a high-dose oestrogen form of HRT then progesterone cream alone may not adequately protect the endometrium from hyperplasia, which can lead on to cancer. If this is the case for you, then discuss with your gynaecologist why you are on a high-dose oestrogen and see about switching. Often only a low dosage of oestrogen is needed to relieve symptoms, then the supplementary progesterone cream can do its work and protect the endometrium so that the hyperplasia which can lead to cancer will not occur.

You might also find it helpful to read the section on cancer and natural progesterone on page 109.

I HAVE BEEN USING NATURAL PROGESTERONE FOR SOME TIME WITH GOOD RESULTS. RECENTLY I HAVE DEVELOPED DRYNESS OF THE VAGINA AND MY DOCTOR SAYS I MUST TAKE HRT FOR THIS.
This is an unpleasant symptom but it does not justify taking HRT without first trying some other methods. For a dry vagina you can use your natural progesterone cream locally, or take vitamin E capsules, both by mouth and applied directly to the vagina. To use locally, simply cut the top off a capsule and squeeze the oil in, or apply it with your fingers. There are also quite a few specific vaginal lubricants, many plant-based, available in your local health store. Talking to a homoeopath or herbalist would also be helpful.

I HAVE TRIED MOST THINGS TO COUNTERACT A DRY VAGINA,
BUT NOTHING HAS WORKED. MY DOCTOR SAYS THAT I CANNOT
USE OESTROGEN VAGINALLY ON ITS OWN, BUT WILL GIVE ME HRT.
I AM ALREADY TAKING NATURAL PROGESTERONE, SO WHAT ELSE
CAN I DO?

You do not need to take HRT. Certainly the dryness of the
vagina is probably due to a lack of oestrogen, but if you have
no other symptoms of a lack of oestrogen generally, such
as hot flushes or night sweats, then it is quite unnecessary
to take HRT. If alternative methods such as herbs or vitamin
E have not worked for you, then the problem can be treated
locally with a vaginal oestrogen cream. While you will certainly absorb some of the oestrogen from the vaginal cream,
your endometrium, which is probably what your doctor is
worried about, will continue to be protected by the natural
progesterone cream you are using. The safest vaginal creams
contain oestriol alone, or you can also get a tri-oestrogen
formula which contains oestradiol, oestrone and oestriol.
The important thing is not to take any form of oestradiol on
its own, as this is too stimulating to the cells.

SINCE MY MENOPAUSE STARTED I HAVE SUFFERED FROM DRYNESS
OF THE VAGINA. BECAUSE OF A FAMILY HISTORY OF BREAST CANCER
I DO NOT WANT TO USE ANY OESTROGEN. WHAT CAN I DO?

First thing to try could be using natural progesterone cream
directly into the vagina. Many women find this solves the
problem if used initially two or three times a week, then if
the condition improves to use it as and when they feel they
need it. If this does not solve the problem, you could try
a small amount of a vaginal cream which contains only
oestriol, which is the least stimulating of all the oestrogens.
Any of it which you absorb would be balanced by the natural
progesterone cream which you are using, and would be
unlikely to increase your risk of breast cancer.

If you prefer not to take any additional oestrogen at all,

then there are also available specific lubricants which contain no hormones. You could ask your doctor about Replens or Astroglide, which are readily available, or have a look in your local health store as they will carry some natural alternatives based on plant extracts.

WHY DO WE GET HOT FLUSHES AT MENOPAUSE?

The mechanism of hot flushes is not fully understood, but what causes a flush is a disturbance of the temperature control mechanism of the body. The centre which controls this is in the part of the brain known as the hypothalamus. This part of the brain also has areas that control the pituitary, and through it the hormones of the body. There is an area that controls sleep, an area that controls how the body deals with stress, and areas that control the appetite and many other so-called basic bodily functions. It is a common problem for the temperature control mechanism to be upset at the time of menopause, when the levels of oestrogen and progesterone are falling, but they also occur during pregnancy when levels of these hormones are very high.

It seems as if it is the changes and fluctuations in the hormone levels – rather than the levels of the hormones themselves – that cause the disturbance which leads to a hot flush. High dosages of an oestrogen will usually control hot flushes, because at the time of menopause the main cause of hot flushes is fluctuations in oestrogen levels, but this is not the only trigger, and it is high doses of oestrogen that will lead to other symptoms of oestrogen dominance.

WHAT CONTROLS HOT FLUSHES BETTER, NATURAL PROGESTERONE OR OESTROGEN?

Hot flushes are due to changes in the levels of oestrogen and progesterone. They do not necessarily indicate low hormone levels, as it is not uncommon for women to experience hot flushes during pregnancy when levels of oestrogen and progesterone are both very high. The changes in the levels of these hormones lead to an increase in the secretion of Gonadotrophic Stimulating Hormone, which is produced by a part of the brain known as the hypothalamus. This hormone affects the levels of the two pituitary hormones, Follicular Stimulating Hormone and Leuteinizing Hormone. It is not certain whether it is the actual changes in the levels of these hormones or the fact that the temperature control mechanism is also situated in the hypothalamus that causes the hot flushes to occur. It may be that the mechanism is somewhere in the hypothalamus because that is also the stress area of the brain, and most women are only too aware that stress can bring on a hot flush.

Giving high levels of oestrogen will stop hot flushes because this irons out fluctuations in the levels of oestrogen, though this will of course produce other side-effects such as bloating and breast tenderness. Often, the use of phyto-oestrogens will help alleviate hot flushes by enabling the body to use its oestrogen more efficiently.

Progesterone will also alleviate hot flushes without any side-effects, though sometimes the hot flushes will become worse before they disappear.

If the hot flushes are very severe it is sometimes necessary to use a combination of oestrogen and progesterone to start with and gradually reduce the oestrogen until you are just using progesterone.

MY HOT FLUSHES ARE STILL DREADFUL EVEN THOUGH I HAVE BEEN TAKING NATURAL PROGESTERONE FOR SOME MONTHS. AM I NOT USING ENOUGH?

Although many women do get relief from hot flushes after using natural progesterone, it can sometimes make them worse. It can help to understand what causes hot flushes in the first place. They are due to a disturbance in the temperature control mechanism of the body. The centre which controls this is in a part of the brain called the diencephalon and it can be affected by many different things. Changes in oestrogen levels, stress, certain foods (especially spicy ones), caffeine and alcohol are among them. If natural progesterone isn't controlling the flushes after several months of use then there is no point increasing the amount as this is not the answer for you. You might like to consider some alternative ways of dealing with the problem. You will find some suggestions given in the following answers.

NATURAL PROGESTERONE HAS HELPED WITH MY HOT FLUSHES, BUT THEY ARE STILL A NUISANCE. WHAT ELSE CAN I DO?
The first line of attack in trying to alleviate hot flushes is to add in some phyto-oestrogens in the form of herbs such as dong quoi, agnus castus and red sage. Also add some oestrogen-containing foods to your diet, such as soya, tofu, miso, cashew nuts, apples and almonds. Dietary changes alone can often be effective.

Some women find that being under stress seems to be a factor in bringing on the flushes – even worrying you may have a hot flush can sometimes be enough to bring one on. Here it can be helpful to take supplements – vitamin E is effective for flushes, plus an adrenal support mixture to help with the stress (see the Resources chapter).

Often you can identify certain foods or drinks that trigger hot flushes in you – coffee, alcohol and hot or spicy foods are often a problem – then you either have to avoid these items or be prepared to deal with the consequences.

Be as positive as possible about your flushes, and wear layers of clothing so that you can adjust easily to room temperatures. You might also think about carrying a fan, or try one of the neckerchiefs sold in camping shops for keeping cool in summer. They are very popular in hot countries as they contain a gel which expands when the scarf is soaked in cold water. Worn at times of hot flushes it will help keep you cool.

I RESPOND WELL TO HOMOEOPATHIC REMEDIES; ARE THERE ANY
THAT WILL HELP WITH HOT FLUSHES, AS MINE ARE OUT OF
CONTROL?

For some women the homoeopathic remedies sepia and lach-
esis are very helpful, but it would be more useful to consult
a practitioner so that you can have a remedy specifically for
your constitutional type. Hot flushes are believed by some
complementary therapists to be a result of energy rebalanc-
ing itself in the body, as it has to do at the time of menopause.

The effects of hot flushes are not all negative. It is believed
they may even be useful because they help to destroy malig-
nant cells, which are formed more frequently as we age.

HRT GAVE ME PAINFUL BREASTS AND I HAVE COME OFF IT FOR THAT
REASON. WILL NATURAL PROGESTERONE BE ANY BETTER?

HRT gave you painful breasts because the amount of oestrogen it contained was too high for you. The oestrogen had a
stimulating effect upon the breasts which was not balanced
by any natural progesterone. The artificial progestogens in
HRT only mimic some of the effects of natural progesterone
and do not have the same balancing effect as the natural hormone, nor do progestogens have any protective effect on the
breast. All these are contributory factors to painful breasts;
as natural progesterone does not stimulate the oestrogen
receptors you should not have the problem when taking it.

IF OUR PROGESTERONE LEVELS ARE SUPPOSED TO DROP AT
MENOPAUSE WHEN WE STOP OVULATING, SURELY IT CANNOT BE
NATURAL TO SUPPLEMENT WITH IT?

When you stop ovulating your levels of both oestrogen and
progesterone drop quite naturally. This is perfectly normal,
and if you have no symptoms of oestrogen dominance and
your hormone levels are balanced then you will feel fit
and well and not suffer from any of the well-recognized
menopausal symptoms. If this is indeed the case then cer-

tainly it would be unnecessary and unnatural to supplement with progesterone. Sadly, for many women these hormone levels are not in balance, and the huge amounts of excess oestrogen present throw this balance out. Additional progesterone is needed to counteract the effects of the extra oestrogens, particularly if a woman is on HRT or other drug treatments, and lives with pollution – as most of us do.

MY MENOPAUSE HAS JUST STARTED BUT I DON'T HAVE ANY SYMPTOMS. IF I TAKE NATURAL PROGESTERONE NOW, WILL IT PREVENT ME GETTING ANY MENOPAUSAL SYMPTOMS LATER?

Natural progesterone is a hormone and should only be taken when needed, and in the dose stated, for any particular condition. It is not a preventative treatment, and no practitioner experienced in the use of natural progesterone would suggest using it just because you have reached menopause. This is very different from HRT use, which is often recommended to women as a 'preventative' treatment for menopause, though again it ought not to be prescribed in that way.

I FINISHED MY MENOPAUSE SOME YEARS AGO. WILL NATURAL PROGESTERONE MAKE MY PERIODS START AGAIN?

If you have truly finished your menopause then using natural progesterone will not make your periods restart. Periods occur because the endometrium – the lining of the uterus – is built up. This is done by oestrogen, and once your levels of oestrogen have dropped to normal post-menopausal levels the lining will not build up and you will not have any periods. Natural progesterone does not have any effect on building up the endometrium. However, if you have only just stopped having periods, or they occur only once or twice a year, then they may become more frequent when you start using natural progesterone. This is because there is still enough oestrogen to build up the endometrium and the progesterone will have its normal maturing effect on it. So when you stop the natural progesterone for a few days the drop in the level of progesterone will have the normal effect of shedding the endometrium as a period.

MY DOCTOR TELLS ME THAT NOW I AM MENOPAUSAL I AM MORE LIKELY TO HAVE A HEART ATTACK BECAUSE I NO LONGER HAVE THE PROTECTION OF OESTROGEN.

Certainly it is fairly unusual for pre-menopausal women to have heart attacks. During and after menopause it is more common – in fact it is the greatest single cause of death in this age group. However this is not entirely because we lack oestrogen. Men and women do not necessarily have the same type of heart disease. Men tend to suffer from heart attacks because their coronary arteries become blocked and narrowed due to a variety of factors, of which high levels of cholesterol in the diet is an important one. Over the years, the lumen on the artery can become so narrowed with deposits that not enough blood can pass to the heart muscle and a heart attack occurs. There will often have been warnings that this may happen. When a man exercises, the heart needs more blood; there will be a time when there is enough blood going through when resting but not enough when exercising. The result will be the man will experience pain when exercising, and if sensible will pay attention to it.

In post-menopausal women, however, although we can have narrowing of the arteries and a build-up of deposits, it is much more common for the cause of a heart attack to be spasm of the coronary arteries. For this type of heart disease – which affects the majority of women – then oestrogen in the form of HRT will not protect you. Research has been done which suggests that HRT may in fact aggravate coronary artery spasm, where natural progesterone will relieve it.

If your heart disease is due to narrowing of the arteries, then it has been shown that oestrogen does have an effect in preventing the build-up of deposits, but attention to diet can be beneficial.

HOW CAN NATURAL PROGESTERONE HELP WOMEN WITH HEART DISEASE?

In 1997 some research was done in England which showed that progesterone is effective in relaxing coronary arteries which have gone into spasm, and that excess oestrogen can in fact cause spasm. As most menopausal women's heart attacks are due to heart spasm this is obviously an important factor in demonstrating the protective role of progesterone in preventing potentially fatal heart attacks. At the time of publication of this book, most of the research evidence has been obtained from tests on rabbits and monkeys, but some research has been done using women on different combinations of oestrogen, progesterone, progestogens and nothing at all. Although this has only been a small trial, it seems to support the view that progesterone helps to prevent coronary spasm which can lead to a fatal heart attack.

If you are at risk from heart disease then taking natural progesterone would be a very sensible precaution to protect your heart from spasm.

I AM TOLD THAT HRT WILL PROTECT ME FROM HEART DISEASE. WILL NATURAL PROGESTERONE DO THIS AS WELL?

First of all, two things should be realized. One is that while the incidence of heart disease does increase after menopause, it is not as dramatic as many people believe. Secondly, it has not been shown conclusively that HRT does prevent heart disease after menopause – the research on this does not stand up in the opinion of many practitioners.

There are many more factors involved in being prone to a heart attack than a lack of oestrogen. Factors that predispose us to heart attacks include weight problems, having high cholesterol levels and lack of exercise as well as increasing age itself. HRT is a potent medication with well-recognized side-effects such as weight gain and raised blood pressure, so you may want to consider the wisdom of taking it to prevent a disease that you may not even get.

WHY SHOULD USING NATURAL PROGESTERONE ON ANIMALS MEAN IT WOULD WORK FOR ME?
Animal trials have long been used to test various drugs, but it is important that there is some relevance between the animal used for the trial and the condition being treated in the human. The progesterone trial for test of coronary spasm was done on monkeys; this is important because a monkey's heart functions in much the same way as a human's does – monkeys are susceptible to heart disease and they can have heart attacks. Most of the work done in relation to traditional HRT and its ability to prevent heart attacks in post-menopausal women has been done on pigs, and while the pig heart is anatomically very similar to the human, it functions differently. Pigs in fact cannot have heart attacks.

I AM POST-MENOPAUSAL AND MY SKIN HAS RECENTLY STARTED TO LOOK OLD AND THIN. MY DOCTOR SAYS I SHOULD TAKE OESTROGEN, BUT WOULD TAKING NATURAL PROGESTERONE HELP ME?
While it is generally believed that oestrogen makes the skin look younger, this is not actually true. Oestrogen in fact makes the skin thinner. Wrinkles often disappear because oestrogen makes you retain fluid and that can puff up the skin so the appearance of wrinkles is lessened, but you could also have a puffy face and a problem with fluid retention. On the other hand, it has been shown that progesterone will thicken and improve the appearance of old skin. It does not have this effect on young skin, so the mechanism of how it does this must in some way be related to enabling old cells to die off and new ones to regenerate.

DOES NATURAL PROGESTERONE HAVE A GENERAL ANTI-AGEING EFFECT?

There is no scientific basis for this, but in looking logically at how progesterone acts in the body it certainly seems as if it should. We know that ageing of all tissues occurs when there is a slowing down of the process of tissue cell regeneration. The cells of all the tissues of our body have a predetermined life span, at the end of which they should die and be removed by scavenger cells. This is the time when the body replaces them with young new cells.

As we age, this process of cell death and renewal seems to slow down. The cells actually survive longer, but they are old cells and often do not fulfil their functions as well as they should. This process of dying-off of cells is known as apoptosis, and apoptosis is blocked by a gene known as BCL2. It is interesting to note that this gene is stimulated by oestrogens. Taking oestrogens will thus stop cells from dying off and being replaced by new young cells.

Fortunately there is another gene, P53, which encourages normal cell death. This beneficial gene – P53 – is stimulated by progesterone.

From this information it is reasonable to deduce that if you increase your levels of progesterone by supplementation then you will be encouraging the activity of gene P53. This means that your cells will be turning over rapidly, just as they did when you were young, and this should have a general rejuvenating effect on the whole body. This may explain why many people who take natural progesterone say they feel generally so much better than they did before.

I AM ON MEDICATION FOR AN UNDERACTIVE THYROID. CAN I USE NATURAL PROGESTERONE, OR WILL THE TWO MEDICATIONS CONFLICT?

You are right to be cautious with regard to combining natural progesterone with thyroid-stimulating drugs. Hypo-thyroidism is often diagnosed at or around menopause, when in actual fact the real problem is one of oestrogen dominance. For a number of years prior to menopause we stop ovulating on a regular basis, and even when we do ovulate we rarely produce much progesterone in the second half of the cycle. As a result, oestrogen dominance occurs. When the body is oestrogen dominant it seems unable to use the thyroid hormone produced by the thyroid in an effective manner. As a result, more thyroid hormone is called for by the body; this results in the pituitary secreting more thyroid-stimulating hormone. It is the rise in the level of this hormone that is often used when making a diagnosis of hypothyroidism.

When you commence supplementing with natural progesterone you will in effect reverse the situation of oestrogen dominance, and your body will be better able to use the available thyroid hormone your thyroid is making. As a result, you will probably need to reduce or even stop taking your thyroid tablets. It would be best to discuss this with your own doctor, who can then help you to monitor the changes that will occur.

I HAVE HYPERTHYROIDISM. COULD NATURAL PROGESTERONE REPLACE MY MEDICATION?
It is important to remember that using progesterone to correct oestrogen dominance enables the thyroid hormone to work more efficiently. If you need natural progesterone supplementation for any reason you must make sure that your doctor knows and monitors your thyroid activity and can adjust the dosage of your medication if necessary.

SINCE MY PERIODS STOPPED I HAVE NOTICED THE APPEARANCE OF
HORRIBLE THICK HAIRS APPEARING ON MY CHIN. I REMEMBER MY
GRANDMOTHER HAD THIS PROBLEM AND IT BECAME QUITE
SEVERE. CAN I PREVENT THIS HAPPENING TO ME BY USING
NATURAL PROGESTERONE?

The fact that you say your grandmother had the same problem suggests that there could be a genetic or ethnic origin
for your facial hair as opposed to just the hormonal changes
at menopause. The use of natural progesterone may well prevent, or at least improve, this condition because for most
women it seems to appear at the time when progesterone
levels are very low.

WILL PROGESTERONE HELP IMPROVE MY CONCENTRATION AND
MEMORY?

Practitioners who are familiar with progesterone and many
women who have used it will tell you that progesterone
has quite a marked effect upon both concentration and memory. Do bear in mind, though, that lack of memory and
concentration is not always due to hormone imbalance.
Other important factors could be poor nutritional intake,
other medical conditions or medication, stress, fatigue,
depression, lack of motivation or even boredom. All these
will have an effect, and it could also just be that as we get
older we have absorbed much more information and have
lots more things to remember.

CAN PROGESTERONE HELP WITH FATIGUE?

Fatigue can be due to many factors, especially in women of
menopausal age.

It is important to ensure that you have a good diet with
adequate nutrition. Also it is important to check that you are
not anaemic. Slightly heavy periods over a long time can lead
to quite severe anaemia due to lack of iron. If the fatigue is
due to oestrogen dominance – which can cause fatigue both

directly and by causing hot flushes which disturb sleep – then progesterone will help. If it is due to some other cause then you will have to do some investigating to find out exactly what the root of it is. An alternative practitioner may be of help here; you will find some suggestions in the Resources chapter.

IS THERE ANY PROOF THAT NATURAL PROGESTERONE IS BETTER THAN HRT FOR MENOPAUSE?

Practitioners who work with progesterone, and many of the women who use it, will tell you it works from personal experience. In addition there is considerable international research which shows that it works for specific conditions – and there is no research that shows that it does not work.

Having said that, however, some women who use it may find that it does not resolve the problems for which they take it, whether they be hot flushes, tender breasts, vaginal dryness or any other menopausal symptoms. This is because no medication will work for everybody and 'proof' is a very subjective thing. Because there is no evidence of any side-effects when natural progesterone is used in physiological doses, the best advice is simply to try it for yourself.

WHY ARE PROGESTOGENS IN HRT NOT AS GOOD AS NATURAL PROGESTERONE?

Because progesterone is the hormone naturally made in your body and supplementary natural progesterone cream is recognized by your body as identical to the progesterone it produces itself. Progestogens are synthetic, manufactured compounds which can only mimic some of the actions of the true hormone, and have none of its protective effects against cancer, osteoporosis or heart disease.

Progestogens can also have considerable side-effects of their own. It has also been shown that at least one of the progestogens not only nullifies the beneficial effects of oestrogen, but also ensures maintained coronary artery spasm in those cases where it has been induced in progesterone-deficient states. Not good news for women who are concerned about heart disease.

I HAVE BEEN TOLD THAT HRT WILL PROTECT ME FROM ALZHEIMERS AND THAT NATURAL PROGESTERONE WILL NOT. IS THIS TRUE?
There is no clear evidence that HRT protects against Alzheimers disease. There was a study which suggested that a group of women who had taken HRT had less incidence of this disease than a group who had not taken HRT. However, factors such as family history and lifestyle were not considered. Alzheimers, while being a condition one would wish to avoid if at all possible, is statistically not that common; taking a powerful drug to prevent a condition you may not get when there is no evidence as to its effectiveness is not to be recommended. And there is no evidence that natural progesterone would offer any protection, either.

I HAVE HAD MY MENOPAUSE AND FEEL VERY WELL. MY BONE DENSITY SCAN SHOWS NO PROBLEMS, BUT MY ALTERNATIVE HEALTH PRACTITIONER HAS TOLD ME THAT I SHOULD USE NATURAL PROGESTERONE TO PREVENT ANY FUTURE PROBLEMS. WHAT DO YOU THINK?
If you feel well and have no problems which could relate to a lack of progesterone, then you certainly should not supplement with it. Natural progesterone is a hormone, and hormones are powerful substances which should be treated with respect and not used unnecessarily by people who do not need them. This applies to all forms of hormone supplementation and treatment. Hormones should only be taken when needed, in the dose needed, and for as long as needed. No practitioner experienced in the use of natural progesterone would suggest using it just because you have reached menopause.

**I HAVE VARICOSE VEINS. MY DOCTOR SAYS I SHOULD NOT TAKE HRT
BECAUSE OF THIS. CAN I USE NATURAL PROGESTERONE?**

Certainly it is better not to take HRT if you already have
varicose veins. The high oestrogen levels could make
your varicose veins worse because oestrogen interferes with
the muscular tone in blood vessels. Also, oestrogen increases
the risk of blood clotting. If blood is flowing slowly, or even
being stagnant in a varicose vein it is more likely to clot than
normal. Progesterone, on the other hand, improves the tone
of blood vessels and regulates the blood-clotting mecha-
nisms.

**I HAVE IRRITABLE BOWEL SYNDROME. WILL NATURAL
PROGESTERONE HAVE ANY EFFECT ON IT?**

This is a very variable condition from one person to another.
If you find that your symptoms have become worse since you
entered menopause, then it may well be that supplementation with natural progesterone could help. Progesterone is a
muscle relaxant, and if you have bowel spasm associated
with oestrogen dominance then progesterone should help to
relax it.

**I AM TAKING CORTICO-STEROIDS FOR MY JOINTS. CAN I TAKE
NATURAL PROGESTERONE AS WELL?**

There is no reason at all why you should not take natural
progesterone as well as your cortico-steroids. In fact it would
be a sensible thing to do, because it seems that taking
cortico-steroids can produce oestrogen dominance in some
women, and progesterone could balance this. Also if you are
taking cortico-steroids you are increasing your risk of osteoporosis, and progesterone will certainly help you continue
to build up bone.

I HAVE AN INFLAMMATORY CONDITION OF MY JOINTS. MY DOCTOR HAS SUGGESTED CORTICO-STEROIDS BUT I AM NOT HAPPY TO TAKE THEM. COULD NATURAL PROGESTERONE HELP?

It is quite possible that supplementation with natural progesterone could help your joints if the condition is due to an inflammatory process because progesterone has some anti-inflammatory properties. If you are not happy taking the steroids, then it would be worth trying progesterone first to see if you do get a benefit.

CHAPTER 5

Cancer

Cancer is a word that strikes dread and fear into most people's hearts. For women the most feared cancer is probably breast cancer, followed closely by ovarian, endometrial and cervical cancers.

The incidence of breast cancer is increasing rapidly. Fifty years ago the risk of breast cancer was 1 in 50, now it is nearer to 1 in 8. These cancers are almost always oestrogen-responsive and are rich in oestrogen receptors which cause proliferation of breast tissue when exposed to oestrogen. Oestrogen levels may be higher than normal for the body as a result of oestrogen dominance due to a lack of progesterone, taking the Pill, HRT, or from external environmental oestrogen. It is also thought that exposure to abnormally high oestrogen from any source when in the womb can sensitize breast cells and make them more responsive to oestrogen in later life.

There is a considerable amount of scientific evidence available which indicates that progesterone protects against breast cancer. Research has shown that survival rates following surgery for breast cancer are much better if women have surgery at a time when their progesterone levels are high. Survival rate is also better in women with high levels of progesterone than those with low levels. It is rare in women who have a normal oestrogen/progesterone balance throughout their lives.

It is so easy for a woman to increase her progesterone levels by using natural progesterone cream that if there is any risk of breast cancer because of family or other factors, or if she already has breast cancer, then she should do so.

Endometrial or uterine cancer is also an oestrogen-stimulated cancer. Traditional HRT contains oestrogen and a progestogen to protect the uterus from over-stimulation and the development of pre-cancerous cells (hyperplasia). Sometimes, however, if the oestrogen levels in HRT are very high this hyperplasia will occur in spite of the progestogen. If this happens, hysterectomy is often recommended. It is a great pity to have what may be unnecessary major surgery when reducing oestrogen or supplementing with sufficient natural progesterone would solve the problem.

Cervical cancer does not seem to be so directly linked to oestrogen dominance. There is still probably a link, as being on the Pill certainly increases the risk. Other risk factors are smoking, multiple partners and human papilloma wart virus infection.

Ovarian cancer is often described as a silent cancer because it is difficult to diagnose and can be well advanced before a diagnosis is made. It is this fear of ovarian cancer that prompts many surgeons to insist on removing the ovaries when they do a hysterectomy. The reason given is to protect a woman from cancer, and the oft-quoted phrase is 'because you don't need your ovaries any more now, do you?' What tends to be forgotten is that ovarian cancer is a fairly rare cancer and that the ovaries continue to have a hormonal role after menopause. Because the diagnosis of ovarian cancer is difficult, then women who are at risk should consider routine screening. This consists of a combination of a specific blood test for ovarian cancer antigen and regular pelvic examinations and scans. The following list may help you identify if you are at risk.

Risk factors for ovarian cancer:

- past or present oestrogen dominance
- having used fertility drugs
- family history
- nulliparty – never having been pregnant.

It is thought that the development of all cancers may be precipitated, or made worse by, high oestrogen levels. This is because the effect of oestrogen on almost all cells is to stimulate growth.

The effect of progesterone is to counteract this stimulation of the cells. We also know that the process of tissue renewal is affected by both oestrogen and progesterone. Cells should reach a certain age, die and be replaced by new ones. If they do not, then the old cells change and may become cancerous. Oestrogen prevents this dying off of cells, thus encouraging old cells to remain and become cancerous. Progesterone, on the other hand, encourages the cells to die and to be renewed. Thus we can see that oestrogen dominance may well play a significant part in all cancers, not just those that are specific to women.

Cancer: Questions and Answers

I HAVE ENDOMETRIAL CANCER, CAN NATURAL PROGESTERONE HELP?

Endometrial cancer is caused by an excess of oestrogen. This can either be because the oestrogen that the body naturally produces is not being balanced with enough production of progesterone, or because oestrogen is being given to the woman without the protection of either natural progesterone or artificial progestogens.

It would not be wise to consider the use of progesterone as a sole treatment of endometrial cancer, as there is no evidence to suggest that it can reverse the cancer once it has started. Progesterone will, however, protect the endometrium from cancer and certainly ought to be considered as a protective and preventative measure against further cancer developing.

MY GYNAECOLOGIST HAS TOLD ME THAT IF I USE OESTROGEN WITH A PROGESTERONE CREAM FOR FIVE YEARS I WILL INCREASE MY RISK OF ENDOMETRIAL CANCER FOURFOLD. IS THIS TRUE?
This is a very sweeping and misleading statement because it does not take into account how much oestrogen you are taking, nor how much progesterone cream you are using. Furthermore, it suggests that the combination of oestrogen and progesterone cream increases the risk of endometrial cancer, which is definitely untrue. Certainly long-term use of oestrogen on its own will increase your risk of endometrial cancer, but even that is unlikely to increase it fourfold.

Originally HRT consisted of just oestrogen, and endometrial cancer did occur in a number of women. In order to protect the uterus from the oestrogen, a progestogen – an artificial chemical which mimics some of the actions of progesterone – was added to the HRT. The use of the progestogen ensured a monthly bleed, which prevented the lining of the uterus from building up and becoming cancerous. With traditional HRT, because of the high dosages of oestrogen used, this increase in the lining of the uterus can still occur even when progestogens are used. The result of this is the condition known as endometrial hyperplasia, and its existence is often used as a reason for performing a (probably unnecessary) hysterectomy.

While it has been shown that natural progesterone can protect the endometrium against the stimulating effects of extra oestrogen, if you are using oestrogen in the high dosages normally associated with traditional HRT then progesterone cream may not adequately protect the endometrium from hyperplasia. However, if a low dosage of oestrogen, which is often all that is needed to relieve symptoms, is being taken then progesterone cream can protect the endometrium and hyperplasia of the endometrium (which can lead to cancer) will not occur.

CAN TAKING PROGESTERONE CAUSE BREAST CANCER?
Progesterone never causes breast cancer. If a breast cancer is described as being progesterone-sensitive it does not mean that the progesterone caused the cancer, or that the administration of progesterone will make it recur. What it means is that the breast cancer has receptors that are sensitive to progesterone.

The effect of progesterone on the breast is to reduce proliferation of the tissues, and it is this proliferation that makes cancer more likely. So by using progesterone you are positively protecting your breasts against the risk of cancer.

If oestrogen is given on its own as a form of HRT, as it was in the 1960s and early 1970s, it can cause cancer of the lining of the uterus. This is the reason that oestrogen replacement therapy went out of favour and why women should not be prescribed unopposed oestrogen. Current forms of HRT for women who have not had a hysterectomy usually contain some form of artificial progestogen to protect the uterus, although natural progesterone would be a better way to approach the problem.

We have always known that unopposed oestrogen is a major factor in the acceleration of breast cancer. What is now becoming clear from research presented at an international cancer conference in 1998 is that unopposed oestrogen may actually be the cause of some types of cancer. For this reason alone, to give themselves maximum protection women need adequate levels of progesterone to balance out any symptoms of oestrogen dominance.

I HAVE BEEN TOLD THAT NATURAL PROGESTERONE INHIBITS OESTROGEN, SO CAN IT BE USED INSTEAD OF TAMOXIFEN FOLLOWING BREAST CANCER?

It is not true that natural progesterone inhibits oestrogen. Oestrogen and progesterone are female hormones that occur naturally in the body and should occur in quantities that balance each other out. The importance of progesterone is that it balances out the effects of oestrogen. You can see this clearly in the list on pages 4 – 5.

Breast cancer is usually an effect of oestrogen dominance. If this dominance can be counteracted, then the activity of breast cancer cells should be inhibited. It is claimed that tamoxifen does this. However, tamoxifen is a very potent drug (actually a weak oestrogen) with unpleasant side-effects of its own and, in the opinion of many people, is best avoided. On the basis that natural progesterone prevents oestrogen dominance and has no reported or known side-effects, then it is preferable to use natural progesterone instead of tamoxifen for the suppression of oestrogen dominance following breast cancer.

I HAVE HAD A PROGESTERONE-RESPONSIVE BREAST CANCER, SO IS NATURAL PROGESTERONE SAFE FOR ME TO USE?

The breast cells have both oestrogen and progesterone receptors. However, the effect of stimulating these receptors is different. If oestrogen receptors are stimulated they will encourage the breast tissue cells to develop, proliferate and become more active. This is how cancers which are oestrogen-receptor positive can develop and spread. If progesterone receptors are stimulated they will have a different effect on the cells: to counteract the stimulating effects of oestrogen. This will prevent the proliferation and spread of cancer cells.

There has been considerable research done which shows that high levels of progesterone in the body prevent the spread of breast cancer and also increase the likelihood of a good future prognosis for those women with a history of cancer. On this basis, and in discussion with your own doctor and consultant, it most certainly is safe to take natural progesterone.

WHAT IS THE DIFFERENCE BETWEEN USING NATURAL PROGESTERONE AND USING TAMOXIFEN IF YOU HAVE BREAST CANCER?

Natural progesterone counteracts the stimulating effects of oestrogen on tissues such as those in the breast and endometrium, which have both oestrogen and progesterone receptors.

Tamoxifen is an oestrogen blocker for breast tissue. That is to say, it attaches to oestrogen receptors and prevents the body's own oestrogen from acting on them. However, it continues to have true oestrogenic action on other tissues of the body. Tamoxifen is in fact a weak oestrogen, but seems to have two conflicting characteristics. It can act as an antioestrogen to some tissues and as an oestrogen to others.

Current opinion from the US, as reported by Dr John Lee, is that the manufacturers of tamoxifen cannot continue to claim that this drug blocks oestrogen in the breast tissue. Whatever the outcome of this debate, what is quite clear is that tamoxifen does have a considerable number of side-effects, some of which can be fatal.

CAN I USE NATURAL PROGESTERONE AND TAMOXIFEN TOGETHER, AND ARE THERE ANY SIDE-EFFECTS I SHOULD BE AWARE OF?

Yes, you can use natural progesterone and tamoxifen together. Obviously you would discuss any treatment with your doctor. However, given what we know of the beneficial effects of natural progesterone and its protective role against breast cancer, you may wish to give consideration to whether you do need to take tamoxifen as well. The problem with this drug is that it does have serious reported side-effects.

Among these are:

- blood clots in the lungs
- menstrual irregularities
- damage to the cornea and retina of the eye
- depression
- associated with increased risk of endometrial cancer
- may trigger asthma and liver disease
- known carcinogen.

It may seem strange that a drug which is used after breast cancer treatment should be a known carcinogen, but tamoxifen is listed as a cancer-causing drug by the World Health Organization. Tamoxifen produces this carcinogenic effect by binding with DNA material in the body. There have been reported cases of both endometrial and liver cancer from its use. Until it becomes clear that tamoxifen really does prevent the occurrence and recurrence of breast cancer, it remains a drug that should only be taken with caution bearing in mind its possible side-effects.

Natural progesterone, however, does not have any reported side-effects after more than 25 years of use throughout the world. It is known to have the effect of dampening down the stimulating effect of oestrogen on breast tissues – and this is exactly what you wish to achieve to give yourself maximum protection against the possibility of breast cancer.

I HAVE BREAST CANCER AND AM DUE FOR SURGERY. COULD NATURAL PROGESTERONE HELP ME BEFORE I GO INTO HOSPITAL?
Work has been published that shows that women being operated on for breast cancer who have high levels of progesterone, both at the time of surgery and afterwards, show dramatically improved survival rates. From this point of view, wherever possible women should try to schedule any

surgery in the second half of their menstrual cycle when the progesterone level is highest.

The 30-year retrospective study done at John Hopkins University in the US found that women who were low in progesterone had 5.4 more times more incidence of breast cancer and 10 times more deaths from cancer of all kinds. Also, a French study published in the peer journal *Fertility and Sterility* showed that the value of progesterone lies in the fact that it actually slows down the rate at which cell division occurs in the breast ducts.

It would therefore be a very sensible precaution to ensure your surgery is scheduled for the latter part of your menstrual cycle when your progesterone level is normally at its highest. It would also be sensible to supplement with natural progesterone to ensure you've got adequate levels at the time of surgery, and to maintain the progesterone supplementation after it. Dr John Lee has said that of all his own patients treated in this way for breast cancer, none has subsequently died from the disease.

Sources of help for cancer patients are listed in the Resources chapter.

I HAD BREAST CANCER 15 YEARS AGO AND NOW HAVE
OSTEOPOROSIS. I BELIEVE I CAN'T HAVE HRT, SO WHAT ELSE CAN I
DO?
No, you will not be prescribed HRT as you would be a prime risk for further cancer if you were to be given it. However, there is still a great deal that can be done to help your osteoporosis. Taking natural progesterone will enable you to build up new bone and will further be protective against any further breast cancer risk. Reading the following chapter on osteoporosis will also be helpful for you.

I AM WORRIED ABOUT TAKING ANY SUPPLEMENTS WHICH MIGHT
STIMULATE MY BREAST CANCER TO START UP AGAIN.
Natural progesterone will not increase the risk of a recurrence of your breast cancer as taking HRT can do. Women
with high levels of progesterone have actually less risk of a
recurrence of breast cancer than women with low levels do.

CAN USING NATURAL PROGESTERONE PREVENT OTHER CANCERS?
There has not been enough work done in this field to answer
this question with any degree of authority. However what is
known is this: The body is constantly renewing its cells. All
cells have a predetermined lifetime after which they should
die, be removed and replaced by the body with new, young,
healthy cells. For some reason not understood sometimes
this does not happen and the old cells remain and begin to
function and grow in an abnormal way which is known as
cancerous. There is a gene (BCL2) which blocks the process
that tells cells when it is time to die. This gene is stimulated
by oestrogen. As a result it is more active when oestrogen is
dominant.

If supplementation with natural progesterone is used this
will reduce the oestrogen dominance and as a result stop or
slow down the activity of this gene. In addition to gene BCL2
there is another gene (P53) which encourages the cells to
know it is time to die. This gene is actually stimulated by
progesterone. As a result of supplementing with natural
progesterone this gene will be made more active.

See also Chapter 2, page 24.

CHAPTER 6

Osteoporosis

INTRODUCTION

Osteoporosis, or brittle bone disease as it is sometimes called, is a condition most women fear. While it is certainly an unpleasant and dangerous condition, it is not as common as we are led to believe. It's important to remember that it certainly does not affect all women at menopause. The major problem is that there are no warning signals, and even when the bone has been considerably weakened by osteoporosis it is virtually impossible to tell if you are suffering from this condition. Again, this has led to it being commonly referred to as 'the silent killer'.

Another common fallacy about osteoporosis is that doctors can tell from looking at you, or from ordinary x-rays, whether or not you have it. This is simply not possible. There are only two ways in which osteoporosis can be diagnosed: one is when a bone fractures in response to a relatively minor degree of trauma, and the other is by having a bone density scan. It is for this reason that if you have any lifestyle risk or family history of this disease, your doctor should give you a bone scan to assess your vulnerability.

THE NORMAL LIFE CYCLE OF
OUR BONES

Bone is a living tissue, and like all other living tissue in our bodies is constantly being renewed throughout our lives. Bone is built up by cells called osteoblasts, and broken down by another set of cells called osteoclasts. Our bone density at any time is the result of the balance between these two processes. When we are young and growing, we build up bone faster than we break it down. During much of our adult life the two processes are in balance and our bone density remains static. If our hormones remain in normal balance by the time we reach our thirties, it is then that the process of breakdown begins to slightly overtake the rate at which we are building bone and bone density begins to fall by about 1 per cent a year.

For three or four years at the time of menopause, due to changes in hormone balance this rate increases in women so that during this specific time we are losing roughly 3 per cent of our bone density per year. After this, the hormone balance is reset and the loss of bone density then reverts back to just 1 per cent a year again. This loss of bone is normal, as generally older people are not as active as they were when younger and do not need such heavy bones.

Healthy Bones

The maintenance of good bone structure and density relies upon many factors. These include the adequate presence of certain hormones, how good your diet is, lifestyle factors and whether you take any weight-bearing exercise. It is possible to make a reasonable assessment of your risk for osteoporosis by analysing these various factors and their relative importance to you. This is quite a long list, and obviously some factors have a greater degree of importance than others.

Nutritionally there is a great deal that can be done to help if you have osteoporosis, or are at risk from it. You will find supplement and diet suggestions among the questions beginning on page 127.

KNOWN RISK FACTORS FOR OSTEOPOROSIS

family history of the disease
poor general diet – this also means having too much fat and protein
disturbed eating patterns which have resulted in anorexia or bulimia
lack of nutrients – specifically calcium, magnesium, boron, vitamins D and C and other trace minerals
smoking
alcohol
lack of exercise
contraceptive pill
nulliparity (not having any children)
late puberty
early menopause
severe oestrogen deficiency
progesterone deficiency
parathyroid imbalance
lack of calcitonin

Oestrogen versus Progesterone

The argument that oestrogen is the important hormone to prevent bone loss looks suspect when you realize that the breakdown of bone is often seen to increase in women who are in their thirties, when they are still menstruating and have normal levels of oestrogen.

The hormone which is beginning to decrease in a woman in her thirties is in fact progesterone. This may be occurring because in spite of having regular, or fairly regular, periods she is no longer ovulating and therefore not producing any progesterone. Even if she is ovulating most months, the surge of progesterone which occurs after ovulation is not maintained. This condition is very common and is known as luteal phase progesterone deficiency.

Progesterone has a direct effect upon the cells which build up new bone and stimulates them to begin the process of building new layers. For this reason alone, if you have osteoporosis or a tendency towards it, then taking natural progesterone would be a sensible safeguard. This new bone built up by progesterone is strong, not aged. This is directly contrary to oestrogen, which will only slow down the breakdown of bone and preserves your old bone for longer, but it is not producing any new bone. In fact oestrogen only has this effect of slowing down bone loss for a limited number of years (estimated at between six and eight), and for only as long as you continue taking it. When you stop taking oestrogen, much of the bone which has been preserved is recognized by the body as old bone and is rapidly broken down. This can leave your bones as bad or worse than they were before you started taking the oestrogen.

Osteoporosis: Questions and Answers

I AM ON THE CONTRACEPTIVE PILL TO HELP MY OSTEOPOROSIS.
WOULD NATURAL PROGESTERONE BE BETTER?
The reasoning behind giving you the contraceptive pill to stop your osteoporosis from becoming worse is that, by giving you extra oestrogen, the osteoclasts which break down bone will not be so active. While this may prevent the excessive breakdown of bone, it will only do so while you continue to take it. If at any time you stop taking the Pill, then

the bone which has been retained, which is very old bone, will be removed fairly quickly and you will be no better off than when you started. Also, there is some doubt about the Pill's ability even to have this action, as it does not contain a natural oestrogen.

What is more important with regard to osteoporosis is that new bone is built up by the osteoblasts. There is only one hormone that will stimulate the osteoblasts and build up more bone, and that hormone is progesterone. Certainly no synthetic hormone or drug has this action.

I AM ON THE PILL BOTH FOR CONTRACEPTION AND TO HELP MY OSTEOPOROSIS. AS I AM ONLY IN MY THIRTIES, WILL I NOT BE PRODUCING ENOUGH NATURAL PROGESTERONE OF MY OWN?

While you are on the Pill your ovulation will be suppressed. As a result of this, the progesterone that your body would normally make after ovulation each month will not be produced. You will therefore be producing less progesterone when you are on the Pill than you would do naturally. Thus, while breakdown of bone may be reduced, the build-up of new bone is reduced as well.

If osteoporosis is a major factor, then in order to encourage your bone development you would be better advised to stop the Pill and use some other non-hormonal form of contraception. You will also need to take natural progesterone cream at the suggested dose for osteoporosis prevention in order to help your body to increase your own progesterone levels.

It is also important to remember that in addition to progesterone the osteoblasts also need specific nutrients. You will find these listed in the question on page 127.

IF I STOP TAKING NATURAL PROGESTERONE WILL MY OSTEOPOROSIS BECOME WORSE?

If for any reason you stop taking natural progesterone, the bone that has built up will remain until broken down by natural processes. This is unlike oestrogen, the action of which ceases immediately you stop taking it, leading to the rapid breakdown of bone.

IF YOU HAVE LOST HEIGHT THROUGH OSTEOPOROSIS AND TAKE NATURAL PROGESTERONE, WILL YOU GET YOUR HEIGHT BACK?

If you have lost height as a result of osteoporosis it will be due to the fact that one or more of your vertebrae has collapsed. The use of natural progesterone plus correct diet and exercise will enable you to build up new bone and should prevent the collapse of more vertebra. It should also enable you to build up new bone in the vertebra which has collapsed, but sadly it will not rebuild the vertebra nor restore it to its original shape and size. You will not therefore be able to regain any height you have lost.

All loss of height in old age is not due to osteoporosis. It can also be due to the fact that the discs which exist between each vertebra, cushioning them, become flatter with age.

I AM AFRAID THAT I MIGHT DEVELOP OSTEOPOROSIS WHEN I REACH MENOPAUSE. SHOULD I TAKE NATURAL PROGESTERONE TO PREVENT IT?

It is important to remember that not everyone develops osteoporosis, and it is always unwise to take treatment to prevent a condition you may not develop. There are certain people who would benefit from taking natural progesterone before osteoporosis is fully developed, but that is because they are in a high-risk category.

If you would like to know if you might be affected, these are some of the factors involved:

family history of osteoporosis
small frame or being very thin
early menopause
abnormal absence of menstruation
eating problems
lack of calcium in diet
inactive lifestyle
smoking
drinking alcohol.

I AM SURE I AM AT RISK FROM OSTEOPOROSIS, HOW CAN I TELL?
Osteoporosis can only be accurately diagnosed by having a
bone density scan. It cannot be diagnosed by looking at
someone's build or taking an x-ray. If you feel that you are at
risk, then at or near your menopause you should have a bone
density scan carried out.

If your bone density is normal you have no cause for concern, although it would be sensible to repeat the scan in five
years' time or after your menopause.

If your bone density is a bit on the low side then you
should think of changing your diet and improving your
lifestyle. Then repeat the bone density scan again in three or
four years' time.

If the bone scan shows low density, then certainly one of
the most helpful things you can do is to supplement with
natural progesterone.

THE DOCTOR HAS SUGGESTED I HAVE AN X-RAY TO DIAGNOSE MY
OSTEOPOROSIS. WILL THAT WORK?
No, it is not an accurate way to do this. The density of the
bone shown on a x-ray relates to the strength of the x-rays
used, not the density of the bone. Strong x-rays penetrate the
bone easily and make it look less dense.

If a radiologist makes a diagnosis of osteoporosis from an
x-ray, or even suggests it as a possibility, you must have it

checked further with a bone density scan. These scans use a standard way of measuring the density of your bone and are therefore much more accurate (see resources page 152).

THE CONSULTANT MY DOCTOR SENT ME TO SAYS I HAVE OSTEOPENIA AND HAS RECOMMENDED HRT. IS THIS THE SAME AS OSTEOPOROSIS?
Osteopenia is a term used to indicate you have a tendency to be osteoporotic or are at risk possibly in the future. Unless there has been a bone scan done, you cannot be diagnosed as having either osteopenia or osteoporosis. If you know you are at risk, then natural progesterone supplementation would be the best course of action to protect your bones and prevent osteoporosis from developing.

MY DOCTOR HAS PUT ME ON HRT FOR MY OSTEOPOROSIS AND HAS SAID I SHOULD TAKE IT FOR LIFE. WILL IT PROTECT ME THAT LONG?
Although oestrogen in the form of HRT is often prescribed for long-term – indeed lifelong – usage for osteoporosis, it does not provide the same protection as natural progesterone. Plus there is the little-known fact that when HRT is taken over a number of years the actual effects are not continuously as good, so that the benefit you get in year one is better than that in year six or seven. If for any reason you need to stop taking HRT – for example if you are suffering from side-effects – then the benefits of the slowing down of bone loss are immediately lost and the bone is then extremely vulnerable to fracture. Also the bone is then rapidly broken down by the osteoclasts, which have been held at bay by the oestrogen.

I HAD BREAST CANCER 15 YEARS AGO AND WAS NOT ALLOWED HRT. I NOW HAVE OSTEOPOROSIS. CAN I USE NATURAL PROGESTERONE?
No woman who has breast cancer ought to be given HRT and you were well advised not to take it. Using natural proges-

terone will enable you to build up new bone without any risk to you whatsoever. Your history of breast cancer will not be a problem, as natural progesterone is safe for you to use, and indeed will provide some protection against any further development of secondary cancer in the breasts.

IS IT ENOUGH JUST TO TAKE NATURAL PROGESTERONE TO HELP MY OSTEOPOROSIS?

There are few magic wands in medicine, and it is rarely enough just to do one thing and trust that it will resolve the problem completely. Osteoporosis in particular has many factors which affect it, and although using natural progesterone will be enormously helpful you do also need to look at your diet and make sure you have the correct balance of the right nutrients. There are several osteo supplements on the market to consider adding to your diet, but make sure you also have adequate supplies not just of calcium and magnesium but also of boron and vitamins C and D. A nutritionist will be able to help you with this, and there are excellent suggestions in the books listed in the Resources chapter. Kate Neil and Patrick Holford's book *Balancing Hormones Naturally* is particularly comprehensive.

Regular weight-bearing exercise is important – but try not to get obsessed with the word exercise. Walking, skipping and dancing are all weight-bearing, and if you enjoy these activities they will not seem like 'exercise'. Only you can decide how much effort you want to put in to avoid problems with osteoporosis, but it is important to try and find something you enjoy and will be therefore more willing to do on a regular basis.

IS THERE ANY AGE AT WHICH YOU ARE TOO OLD FOR NATURAL PROGESTERONE TO BE EFFECTIVE FOR OSTEOPOROSIS?

No, your bones continue to be broken down and built up as long as you live, so it is never too late to start taking natural progesterone or gaining the benefit of increased bone density. Indeed, the older you are the more important it is to guard against brittle bones, so do not let age put you off. As natural progesterone has no known side-effects there is no need to be concerned about using it for the rest of your life.

WHAT IS THE CORRECT AMOUNT OF NATURAL PROGESTERONE TO TAKE FOR OSTEOPOROSIS PREVENTION?
It depends on your age and hormone state. But generally there are two categories:

1 If you are pre-menopausal you should be having reasonably regular periods and ovulating regularly. If this is happening you should be producing enough progesterone yourself to prevent osteoporosis and there should be no need to supplement. However, if have a low bone density for your age – shown through a bone scan – ask your doctor to take either a blood or saliva test for progesterone in the second half of your cycle. This will show whether or not you are ovulating and whether or not you are producing sufficient progesterone. If you are ovulating and the hormone levels are normal, then you need to look for other causes of osteoporosis. You may need a medical practitioner to help you do this, as it can be difficult to diagnose. As you are pre-menopausal, you do not want the progesterone supplementation to confuse your ovaries and interfere with ovulation. For that reason you should use approximately 20–30 mg of natural progesterone cream daily from the day on which you would expect to ovulate until the day before you would expect your period to start. Ovulation normally occurs 14 days before your period starts. This is so even if you have a cycle that is longer or shorter than the average.
2 Post-menopausal women do not have to worry about ovulation or fitting in with a menstrual cycle, and they would

use approximately 20 mg of natural progesterone cream. This should be taken daily except for five days each calender month. The reason for this break is to prevent the progesterone receptors from becoming blocked. The simplest way to do this is to 'decide' on an easily remembered time – like the first week or the last week in the month – and use that as your 'free' week. If a post-menopausal woman is only using natural progesterone for osteoporosis, and not for any other menopausal symptoms, then she can use the cream just once a day. If there are other symptoms as well, then it is more effective to split the dose and take it twice a day to maintain steadier blood levels of the hormone.

I HAVE OSTEOPOROSIS AND CANNOT TAKE HRT. MY DOCTOR WANTS ME TO TAKE FOSAMAX (GENERIC NAME: ALENDRONATE SODIUM, A BISPHOSPHONATE). COULD I USE NATURAL PROGESTERONE INSTEAD?

Certainly you could use progesterone. It would stimulate your osteoblasts and, provided you combine it with an intake of all the necessary nutrients and take weight-bearing exercise, you should build up new bone.

Fosamax is an unpleasant drug to take. You have to remain upright after you have taken it for at least half an hour. This is to prevent the drug from eating ulcers – it can even make holes in the wall of your oesophagus. It acts on the osteoclasts and seems to poison them so that they no longer work. As a result, bone breakdown is stopped. They also accumulate in very small amounts in the osteoblasts, but any effect on them is not mentioned in the literature. It seems logical, however, that if they stop the action of the osteoclasts then they may well stop the action of the osteoblasts as well. In any case they act rather like HRT in that they slow the breakdown of bone but do not stimulate the build-up of new bone.

I HAVE BEEN ADVISED TO TAKE DIDRONEL (GENERIC NAME ETIDRONATE DISODIUM, A BISPHOSPHONATE/CALCIUM SUPPLEMENT) AND EXTRA CALCIUM FOR MY OSTEOPOROSIS. WILL NATURAL PROGESTERONE WORK AS WELL?

Progesterone will work better than Didronel to build up your bones, and will do so without any side-effects. Progesterone will stimulate your osteoblasts and they will build up new bone. Didronel, on the other hand, has an effect only on slowing down the breakdown of bone. It often results in the bone which you do have becoming less strong, because some of the minerals leak out of the bone. This is counteracted by giving you large doses of calcium, which can in some people cause kidney stones.

I ONLY HAVE VERY IRREGULAR PERIODS AND HAVE BEEN FOUND TO HAVE OSTEOPOROSIS. I HAVE USED NATURAL PROGESTERONE FOR 18 MONTHS, LOOKED AT MY DIET AND EXERCISED BUT MY BONE DENSITY HAS NOT IMPROVED. WHAT AM I DOING WRONG?

You certainly seem to be doing all the right things to help improve the density of your bone and it must be very disappointing not to see an improvement. You say that you only have very irregular periods. It could be that your oestrogen levels are very low. Oestrogens play a role in the prevention of osteoporosis in that they help to prevent the excessive breakdown of bone. If your oestrogen levels are very low it could be that in spite of the natural progesterone helping to build up your bones, the lack of oestrogen is allowing the bones to break down faster than they are being built up.

In pre-menopausal women it appears that a much higher level of oestrogens is needed to prevent this excessive breakdown than is the case in post-menopausal women. It could be well worth supplementing with a small amount of natural oestrogen as well as the natural progesterone. You would need a practitioner experienced in this field to help you to work out the correct regime for you.

I HAVE HAD A BONE DENSITY SCAN DONE, BUT DON'T UNDERSTAND THE RESULTS.

Bone density scans are quite difficult to interpret. Because of this it sometimes happens that women are told they have severe osteoporosis – which is a frightening thing to be told – when in fact they only have osteopenia.

When bone density is measured, the results are reported in figures and on a chart. For most people it is easier to understand the chart. This usually has a sloping line which falls from left to right. This is the average normal drop in bone density for a woman. The chart is slightly different for a man.

Above and below this 'average' line are two shaded areas which run parallel to it. You will also see a mark on the chart above your age. This indicates your bone density. If the mark is on or above the average line, you have no cause to be concerned. If your mark is in the shaded area below the line, you have a degree of osteoporosis called osteopenia and need to realize that you are below average and at risk. If your mark is below the shaded area, you have osteoporosois and need to do something about it immediately. If your doctor just quotes the figures at you, ask to see the chart.

I HAVE BEEN USING NATURAL PROGESTERONE FOR SOME TIME NOW. WHEN I HAD THE LAST BONE SCAN DONE, MY DOCTOR SAID MY BONE DENSITY IS 2.5 BELOW STANDARD DEVIATION AND THAT THIS IS VERY GOOD. WHAT DOES IT MEAN?

Standard deviation is a statistical term which in simple terms relates to a range of difference, or deviation, from normal which is acceptable and can be considered within normal range. If your reading is outside this range, then it is considered to be abnormal.

The World Health Organization has set a standard in relation to bone density for what is considered to be osteoporosis. If you are more than 2.5 per cent below this range you are classified as having osteoporosis, and it will be reported as more than 2.5 below standard deviation. In other words this is a statistical way of reporting the result and is useful for statisticians worldwide, but usually serves to confuse patients as well as some doctors.

CHAPTER 7

Progesterone for Men

INTRODUCTION

It is often forgotten that progesterone is a hormone that is produced by both men and women. Progesterone levels in men remain fairly constant until they reach their sixties or even seventies. At this time of life there are other hormone changes in a man in addition to the drop in progesterone levels. The levels of testosterone not only drop, but change from a preponderance of testosterone to one of di-hydro-testosterone. The levels of oestrogens also rise. It is not clear whether these hormonal changes are independent of one another or if perhaps the drop in progesterone precipitates the fall in testosterone. What is clear is that adequate progesterone production is essential for men's health and well-being.

MALE HORMONE PATTERN

The male pituitary produces both Follicular Stimulating Hormone (FSH) and Leuteinizing Hormone (LH). When a boy reaches puberty the hypothalamus starts to secrete Gonadotrophic Stimulating Hormone. This acts upon the pituitary, which then starts to secrete FSH and LH. The FSH action results in enlargement of the testes and the production of sperm. The LH acts on the Leydig cells in the testes –

named after the man who discovered them – and these cells produce progesterone. Of the male production of progesterone, some remains as progesterone and some is converted into testosterone. Men also produce oestrogens in their body, both in the testes and in fat cells. Men do produce considerably less progesterone than women – approximately 5 to 15 mg per day – and it is secreted on a regular daily basis. This is very different from women, whose progesterone is secreted in a cyclical manner every month. Just as in women, there is a complex feedback mechanism between the pituitary and its hormones and the testes and its hormones.

Changes in Hormone Balance in Older Men

While it is well recognized that men frequently experience a decrease in sexual activity as they age, it is not clear whether this is due to ageing, a decline in general fitness, a change in hormone levels or some combination of these factors. All women experience menopause and the change in hormonal balance that results, but not all men have changes in their hormone balance. Even when these changes do occur, the age at which men are affected is later than in women and does not happen in all men. When changes do occur they are usually related to a rise in oestrogen levels. This accounts for the feminizing effects sometimes observed in older men, such as developing fatty tissue at the breasts and needing to shave less often. The levels of both progesterone and testosterone drop, and when testosterone levels fall there is often a corresponding rise in di-hydrotestosterone. This is another form of testosterone and seems to have more aggressive effects than testosterone. It may be that this is the cause of prostatic cancer.

The drop in progesterone levels is important. We know that progesterone has a protective effect against the stimulating effects of oestrogen in women. It has the same protective effect in men against the stimulating effects of testosterone and di-hydrotestosterone. It works in men in two ways: first by acting directly upon progesterone receptors which are present in almost every tissue of the body, and secondly by competing for receptors with testosterone.

Although very little research has been done into the effects and role of progesterone in men, it is clear that a whole range of health problems can be addressed using this hormone. The use of supplemental natural progesterone in men is based partly on a knowledge of physiology – that is, the way in which tissues are supposed to function in the body – and experience gained from observing the effect of supplementation on male patients. It may be that future work will show that natural progesterone is as vital a hormone for men as it is for women.

Progesterone for Men: Questions and Answers

CAN MEN BECOME OESTROGEN DOMINANT?

As explained in the introduction, the levels of oestrogen in men's bodies rise as they become older, which is why they may shave less often and can develop fatty breasts. This could be described as an oestrogen-dominant situation, and supplementation with natural progesterone could be beneficial. It should not be forgotten that men are also exposed to the pollutant xeno-oestrogens in the environment and these too can have oestrogen-like effects on men as well as on women. This oestrogen dominance due to pollution is probably the cause of some of the low sperm counts that are not infrequently seen in otherwise fit and healthy men.

MY WIFE USES A NATURAL PROGESTERONE CREAM. IF IT GETS ON MY SKIN WILL IT AFFECT ME?

There is no need for you to worry at all. To start with, the amount of cream that would remain on the surface of your wife's skin after she has rubbed it in would be so small that it is unlikely even to be absorbed by your skin. Secondly, even if you used the same amount of cream directly on your own skin as your wife uses, the amount would only be about 20 mg. It is often not realized that it is normal for men to make between 5 and 15 mg of progesterone in their bodies every day. The extra amount of progesterone your wife uses could not cause any problems for you.

Another point to remember is that progesterone is not a feminizing hormone. That is the role of the oestrogens. While in the uterus all babies, including boys, are subject to very high levels of progesterone.

IS NATURAL PROGESTERONE SUPPLEMENTATION SAFE FOR MEN?

Progesterone is a hormone that is produced normally in the male by his adrenals and testes. It is a precursor of adreno-cortical hormones and testosterone, so you can see that it has a very important role. There has been very little research on the use of natural progesterone supplementation by men, but there have been no reports of side-effects in over 30 years of use by women and certainly there is nothing to suggest that it is unsafe when used in low dosages.

HOW MUCH NATURAL PROGESTERONE IS AN AVERAGE DOSE FOR A MAN?

This will to some extent depend upon why the natural progesterone is being used. The average man produces between 5 to 15 mg of progesterone per day in the body, and when supplementing with the cream it is usual to use a smaller dose than a woman would take. Probably starting off with an eighth- to a quarter-teaspoon once a day would be sufficient for most men.

IF MEN TAKE PROGESTERONE, SHOULD THEY TAKE A BREAK FROM IT EVERY SO OFTEN AS IS ADVISED FOR WOMEN?

In theory it would seem reasonable to use the natural progesterone on a daily basis. In practice, however, it seems to work better if men stop using it for three to five days a month as is advised for menopausal women. It may be that the receptors work better if they are not subjected to a continuous barrage of progesterone cream but are given a chance to rest.

WHAT ARE THE SIGNS OF OSTEOPOROSIS IN A MAN?

For both men and women there are no early warning signs of osteoporosis. Risk factors are the same for both sexes: poor diet, lack of exercise, excessive smoking and alcohol. An additional risk factor for men is having low levels, or a lack of, testosterone. Osteoporosis can only be diagnosed in two ways. One is when a vertebra collapses or a bone fracture occurs as the result of very little trauma or pressure on it. The other is by having a bone density scan.

ARE MEN AFFECTED BY OSTEOPOROSIS IN THE SAME WAY AS WOMEN?

Osteoporosis is a condition in which there is a decrease in bone density. Bone density at any time is a result of a balance between the bone that is being broken down and the bone that is being built up. This process has been studied in considerable detail in women, but not in men. It seems, however, that for men it is a combination of oestrogens, progesterone and testosterone that are necessary for the maintenance of bone density. Oestrogen slows down the breakdown of bone, progesterone stimulates the build up of bone, but it seems as if testosterone is the most important hormone in the maintenance of bone density in men. Here supplementation with natural progesterone may help because progesterone is a precursor of testosterone.

MY HUSBAND FRACTURED HIS ARM PLAYING RUGBY AND HAS BEEN
TOLD HE HAS OSTEOPOROSIS. IS IT TOO LATE TO DO ANYTHING?
No, it is never too late to do anything with regard to osteoporosis. If a fracture has occurred then it can be treated in the
usual way by surgery or by plaster casts. If your husband has
osteoporosis and does nothing, the bone may not mend. If he
starts by looking at his lifestyle, his diet and his hormone
levels, he can improve his bone density and even eliminate
his osteoporosis. It would certainly be worth using some natural progesterone to stimulate the osteoblasts and to help the
production of testosterone.

I HAVE A COLLAPSED VERTEBRA. HOW MUCH NATURAL
PROGESTERONE SHOULD I TAKE TO REBUILD IT?
Sadly, once a vertebra has collapsed there is little that can
be done to that specific vertebra to rebuild it. It would still be
worthwhile considering natural progesterone supplementation, though, because you are obviously at risk, and it could
prevent further damage from osteoporosis which could result
in other bone fractures.

CAN NATURAL PROGESTERONE PREVENT ENLARGEMENT OF THE
PROSTATE?
Enlarged prostate – or benign prostatic hypertrophy to give
it the proper name – is a common condition in middle-aged
and older men. The prostate gland, which is situated at
the base of the bladder, becomes enlarged. As a result of
this there may be difficulty in passing urine. The cause of
this enlargement is not known but it is clearly a part of the
ageing process. Between the ages of 40 and 60 the muscular
tissue in the prostate is replaced by fibrous tissue, and the
lymphatic cells in the prostate increase. These changes
seem to relate to the levels of testosterone; as progesterone
is a precursor to testosterone production, supplementation
could be helpful.

Supplements for prostate conditions, such as those containing the herb saw palmetto, might also be considered.

CAN NATURAL PROGESTERONE PREVENT ENLARGEMENT OF THE PROSTATE BECOMING CANCEROUS?

Benign hypertrophy of the prostate is – as it says – a benign condition. That is to say, it is not cancerous and does not in itself become cancerous. This does not mean that you cannot develop cancer in an enlarged prostate, because you can, but they are two separate conditions. It is important to remember that prostatic cancer can, and usually does, develop in prostates of normal size and without any symptoms until the late stages. This is why men should consider having routine blood tests, which can identify cancer of the prostate in its early stages, once they reach 40 plus. This test is known as PSA or Prostatic Specific Antigen. High levels of this antigen indicate the possibility of prostatic cancer.

I HAVE CANCER OF THE PROSTATE BUT DO NOT WANT SURGERY OR THE DRUGS SUGGESTED BY MY DOCTOR. WHAT ELSE CAN I DO?

Cancer of the prostate is a slow cancer and does not spread rapidly. Because of this it is worth trying less drastic measures than those suggested by your doctor. It is important that you have a blood test done to establish your levels of PSA (Prostatic Specific Antigen) to find out how fast your cancer is growing. A rising level indicates spread of the cancer, whereas a reducing level indicates improvement.

While there has been no specific research done with regard to the use of natural progesterone in the treatment of cancer, there have over the past few years been some interesting reports from patients with prostate cancer which has been diagnosed both by blood tests and biopsy. These patients have found that, as a result of using natural progesterone for about a year, the levels of PSA in their blood have decreased to normal levels.

There has also been a report of a patient who had secondary prostatic cancer of his bones diagnosed and embarked on a course of natural progesterone supplementation. When he returned later to his doctor, the doctor was unable to find the secondary tumours. The mechanism for this apparently beneficial effect of natural progesterone is not clear. It may relate to progesterone being a precursor of testosterone. Men as they get older have a tendency to produce less testosterone and more di-hydrotestosterone, which seems to have an over-stimulating effect on cells. Progesterone could have the effect of neutralizing the di-hydrotestosterone, which would thus help to maintain testosterone levels.

It is also thought that progesterone may have an effect on the genetic coding of some cells, and in this way prevents the development of abnormal cells.

CAN NATURAL PROGESTERONE PREVENT HEART ATTACKS IN MEN,
AS IT IS CLAIMED TO IN WOMEN?
It is important to realize that the mechanism of heart attacks in men and women is very different. The commonest cause of a heart attack in a man is blockage of the coronary arteries with atheroma. This is a substance which is deposited on the walls of the arteries as a result of excess cholesterol and fat in the blood. These deposits roughen the walls of the artery and the blood is slowed down as it passes through. When blood slows down it is inclined to clot. The combination of these deposits and blood clots can block the artery so that it gradually becomes narrowed, in a similar way as our water pipes become furred up when the water is hard. The blocking of the artery is usually a slow process over a longish period and a man will often experience several minor warning attacks.

In women, narrowed coronary arteries are rare, and a heart attack usually occurs because the coronary arteries go into spasm. This can be caused by oestrogen dominance, and this spasm has been shown to be reversible if progesterone is given. In men with atheroma of the coronary arteries it is possible that spasm may occur as well, particularly if their oestrogen levels rise. Because of this it may well be useful for men with signs of oestrogen dominance to supplement with natural progesterone so that if their heart does go into spasm the progesterone will act to relieve the pressure on the coronary arteries.

COULD PROGESTERONE HELP MY FATHER WHO HAS DEMENTIA?

Brain tissue contains more progesterone receptors than any other tissue in the body; this is true for men as well as women. The progesterone receptors are found in their highest concentrations in the area of the brain known as the limbic centre. This is the part of the brain that deals with thoughts and emotions. If this area malfunctions then disturbances of thought and emotion will occur, such as can be seen in dementia. It may be that a lack of progesterone could cause this sort of malfunction. We do know that depression and mood swings in women are sometimes due to a lack of progesterone and can often be relieved by supplementing with natural progesterone. It also seems that some forms of dementia are helped by the use of supplementary progesterone, and because it has no side-effects, it is certainly worth trying.

I AM ONLY 30 AND AM GOING BALD. COULD NATURAL PROGESTERONE STOP THIS LOSS?

Male pattern baldness seems to relate much more to genetic factors than to hormone levels. If this is the cause of your baldness, then it is unlikely that supplementation with natural progesterone would make any difference. In some men, however, baldness does seem to relate to high levels of testosterone. Because progesterone is a precursor of testosterone one might expect that supplementation with natural progesterone would make matters worse. However this does not seem to be the case, and taking additional progesterone will sometimes help to halt and even reverse the balding process. This may be due to the fact that in some tissues testosterone and progesterone compete for receptor sites, and that if the progesterone occupies the site then testosterone cannot have an effect.

You should also get your doctor to check that you are not anaemic and that your iron and ferritin levels are normal. Ferritin is an iron-storage protein and its level reflects the stores of iron in the body. If iron stores are low it can lead to hair loss in both men and women. There are several herbal remedies that could help with anaemia and could well be useful to try.

WE ARE TRYING FOR A BABY AND TESTS SHOW MY PARTNER HAS A LOW SPERM COUNT. COULD NATURAL PROGESTERONE HELP US?

There are a number of causes of low sperm count. Many of these do not relate to hormone levels but to mechanical reasons or as a result of a non-serious current infection or past infections. The best thing is to consult an expert in this field. It would probably be unwise to use natural progesterone because there has been a report where it was noted that the sperm count in fit young men dropped when they were supplementing with natural progesterone, although it rapidly returned to normal when they stopped using it. This was not men who were prescribed natural progesterone for any medical condition, it was simply part of a trial done at a sports college in England to test the effects of progesterone and other substances on the body under stress.

Nutrition is a key factor here, and for advice and natural help with fertility, see the Resources chapter. You may also find some useful information in the following two answers.

I HAVE A LOW SPERM COUNT WHICH MY DOCTOR SAYS RELATES TO HIGH PROLACTIN. HE HAS GIVEN ME SOME BROMOCRIPTINE TO REDUCE THE PROLACTIN LEVELS BUT IT MAKE ME FEEL AWFUL. WOULD NATURAL PROGESTERONE HELP?

This is an interesting question, and rather difficult to answer. It is certainly clear that progesterone supplementation for women can reduce the levels of prolactin – the hormone secreted by the pituitary – so it is reasonable to think that it might do so in men. We also know that an excess of prolactin lowers oestrogen and testosterone in men, which would certainly have an effect on the sperm count. We don't really have enough information to be sure, but a small trial undertaken by fit, healthy young males using natural progesterone supplementation just to see what effect it would have showed that their sperm counts *decreased* while on the treatment. However, their sperm count did return to normal immediately after stopping the supplement.

It could be worth considering using natural progesterone for a short time to reduce the prolactin, and then stopping it as it could well be that once the prolactin level has been lowered it will not rise again. The reason for suggesting this is that it is often not clear why prolactin levels rise, other than as a result of a pituitary tumour, and they often remain down once they have been reduced.

Bear in mind that stress seems to be a big factor in relation to rising prolactin levels, so you could also address this if it is a factor for you.

MY DOCTOR WON'T PRESCRIBE VIAGRA FOR MY HUSBAND, AND WE WONDERED IF NATURAL PROGESTERONE WOULD HELP WITH IMPOTENCE?

Drugs are often the favoured treatment for impotence, which can be difficult to treat because there are so many areas where there might be problems. Viagra is a drug with some use for specific cases of impotence, but does have serious side-effects which your doctor is probably taking into consideration for your husband's specific case. It cannot be given, for instance, to men already on medication for high blood pressure or depression, and there have been several deaths linked to its use.

Physical causes of impotence can relate to side-effects of medication, alcohol or drug use, vascular disease, low testosterone levels, low zinc intake, high cholesterol levels, endocrine disorders like hypothyroidism, and neurological conditions such as Parkinson's disease and multiple sclerosis.

There is no evidence to suggest that impotence relates to low levels of progesterone. It can sometimes relate to low levels of testosterone, and progesterone is a precursor of testosterone so it is possible that supplementation with natural progesterone might help, but supplementation with testosterone would be better. Ask your doctor to consider this possibility, and also look for some alternative help.

In the US there are reports that the Chinese herb *Tribulis terrestris* is effective for both impotence and infertility, and boosts levels of testosterone. Other supplements which are often suggested are damiana, ginkgo biloba, ashwaganda, ginseng, lycopene, arginine, zinc and a good level of essential fatty acids from the diet.

WOULD USING NATURAL PROGESTERONE IMPROVE MY SEX DRIVE?
The hormone that is most responsible for sex drive in the male is testosterone. While progesterone is certainly a precursor of testosterone, there is no evidence to suggest that supplementation with natural progesterone improves sex drive in men. In women natural progesterone can improve sex drive, but this relates to the fact that normally progesterone is secreted in high quantities by a woman at the time of ovulation. This is to aid the survival of the species, as nature wants a woman to have a higher sex drive at that time in order for her to have the maximum chances of conceiving.

Men may find that talking to a nutritionist about diet may be a good first step, as correct nutrient intake, particularly of zinc, can have an effect here.

I AM A MALE TRANSSEXUAL AND HAVE BEEN GIVEN HIGH DOSES OF OESTROGEN PRIOR TO A SEX-CHANGE OPERATION. THE OESTROGEN MAKES ME FEEL NAUSEOUS. COULD NATURAL PROGESTERONE HELP?

Oestrogen is known to produce a feeling of nausea in some people when taken in high doses. The dose which you have been prescribed, and which you will need in order to develop female characteristics, could well be interpreted as high by your body, as it is still to some extent hormonally male. Progesterone has the effect of balancing oestrogen in the body and in so doing does not counteract any of oestrogen's feminizing effects. It could be very helpful for you to supplement with natural progesterone in a cyclical fashion, say three weeks on and one week off. This could help to reduce the nausea and would give you a better hormone balance than oestrogen on its own.

MY WIFE HAD TERRIBLE MOOD SWINGS DURING MENOPAUSE, AND NATURAL PROGESTERONE SEEMED TO HELP HER. SINCE RETIRING I FIND I SUFFER BADLY FROM DEPRESSION AND WONDERED IF IT WOULD ALSO HELP ME?

It is probable that your wife's depression was due to a lack of progesterone, which is why she was helped by the use of natural progesterone. Lack of progesterone is a common cause of depression in women, but there is no evidence that it has the same effect in men. However, it should be remembered that the brain and nervous tissues in men as well as in women have progesterone receptors in their cells. Obviously these receptors are there for some reason, and their stimulation will have some effect.

It is possible that progesterone lack could cause depression in men. If this were the case then supplementation with natural progesterone would help. You could also consult with an alternative practitioner such as a homoeopath or herbalist, who could offer you some other specific remedies. St John's Wort is often suggested as a herbal remedy for depression and is readily available from herbal suppliers or health stores.

Resources

In the US, where the majority of progesterone products are manufactured, it is possible in most states to buy them over the counter in drug stores. There are some regional variations – check by phoning the manufacturer before purchase.

In the UK and some other parts of Europe, progesterone products are only available on prescription, although it is possible to have a personal import of progesterone products for your own use. We suggest that initially you speak to your own doctor, as it is always best to be monitored by your own medical advisor. Although at the time of writing natural progesterone is classed as a natural medicine and does not therefore appear in a drug register, it is possible to have progesterone prescribed on the NHS, depending on the agreement of your doctor, his or her practice, and in some areas the attitude of the local health authority. If your doctor will not prescribe for you, then you can consult another doctor privately or you can import progesterone products for your own use without a prescription.

Menopause Coaching
Tel: 07000 560 878
Or visit *www.creativecatalyst.co.uk*

Anna Rushton is available to work individually with clients,
or to give talks to interested groups on the change and challenge that menopause offers. Emotionally, this can be a very
demanding time and many women have benefited from practical strategies and information developed to help women
cope and face positively this major life transition.

Natural Progesterone Information Service
NPIS
PO Box 24
Buxton
Derbyshire SK17 9FB

Offers packs for women and health professionals containing
articles, list of doctors and basic information on the uses of
natural progesterone. Also research papers on natural progesterone use worldwide. Send 1st class stamp for details.

LFST Foundation
Tel: 020 8948 5968

Dr Helena Waters offers seminars and retreats for women on
health and wellbeing.
    Phone for details of courses and self-help audio and video
tapes on women's hormonal health from PMS to menopause.

PROGESTERONE PRODUCTS

These are some of the principal suppliers of progesterone creams, which contain the levels of progesterone suggested in this book and in the work of Dr John Lee. The dose suggested for normal physiological use is supplied in a cream that provides 900 mg of progesterone in a 2-oz jar or tube.

Neither the authors, nor Dr Lee, recommend any one particular cream.

UK and Europe

Higher Nature
Burwash Common
East Sussex TN19 7LX
Tel: 01435 882880

UK and European Distributors of Pro-Juven progesterone cream.

Wellsprings Trading
PO Box 322
St Peter Port
Guernsey GY1 3TP
Tel: 01481 33370

European distributors by mail order of Serenity for Women progesterone cream. Free booklet sent on request about natural progesterone usage.

Since publication the oestrogenic herbs have been excluded from the Serenity formula

Wellsprings legally supplies the personal import market by mail order - No Doctor's Prescription Required

Wellsprings Trading Ltd
PO Box 322, St Peter Port   **Tel: 01481 233370**
Guernsey   GY1 3TP   **Fax: 01481 235206**
Wellsprings Trading Ltd is an Associate Company of the Health & Science Research Institute Inc

PERSONAL IMPORTS OF PRO-GEST

It is legal to bring progesterone products into the UK for your own use without a prescription provided you buy them abroad, or have them sent directly to you.

N.H.M. Worldwide
European Call Centre
Gortloskey
Donegal
Eire

Phone: Eire 00353 1 4737881 or UK 07000 437225
Information Line: 00353 73 22522

Offers a comprehensive range of Natural Progesterone products including Progest cream and oil, and a vegan-approved product. Also offers a free 40 page information guide to Natural Progesterone and Saliva Testing.

USA

Transitions for Health
621 SW Alder
Suite 900
Portland, OR 97205—3627
Tel: 503 226 1010

The first progesterone cream company and makers of Pro-Gest. Will suggest a doctor in the US from their records.

AIM International
3904 East Flamingo Ave
Nampa, ID 83687
Tel: 208 465 5116

Makers of Renewed Balance progesterone cream.

Health & Science Research Institute Inc.
4251 Spruce Creek Road
Suite IIC
Port Orange, FL 32317
Tel: 800 222 1415 (US only)

Makers of Serenity for Women, a combination progesterone cream which also contains some oestrogenic herbs.

International Health
8704 E Mulberry St
Scottsdale, AZ 85251
Tel: 602 874 1419

Distributors of Ess-Pro 7 progesterone cream, which also contains some aromatic oils.

Kenogen
PO Box 50423
Eugene, OR 07405
Tel: 541 345 9855

Company founded by Ray Peat, who did much of the original development work on natural progesterone. Produces progesterone in a vitamin E oil.

Products of Nature
54 Danbury Road
Ridgefield, CT 06877
Toll free (US only): 800 665 5952

Makers of Natural Woman cream, which uses rosemary extract as the preservative.

TEST PROCEDURES

Harley Place Screening Services
27 Harley Place
London W1N 2PD
Tel: 020 7323 2383

Harley Place Screening provides comprehensive bone metabolism screening for osteoporosis and saliva tests to determine hormone levels – including for osteoporosis. Clients are given a simple, non-invasive, ultrasound procedure using the heel bone and are then given a print out of the results which are explained to them, and can be given to their own GP or consultant.

Kits for urine tests for bone metabolism and saliva testing kits can be provided by post and an analysis sent direct to the client. Leaflets are also available for a small charge on the use of natural progesterone for specific hormonal imbalance such as PMS, infertility, menopause and osteoporosis.

Harley Place Screening can also arrange medical appointments with Dr Shirley Bond, and also for osteoporosis evaluation. Patients who are unable to travel to London may also have a telephone consultation with her, after filling in a comprehensive questionnaire. Please telephone Harley Place Screening for full details.

You may also contact:
ZRT Laboratory
12505 NW Cornell Road
Portland
OR 197229JRL
Tel: 503 469 0741
Fax: 503 469 1305

USEFUL ADDRESSES

The Nutri Centre
7 Park Crescent
London W1N 3HE
Tel: 020 7436 5122

Shop stocks wide range of nutritional supplements, also available by mail order.

Dandelion Natural Foods
120 Northcote Road
London SW11
Tel: 020 7350 0902

Have an excellent range of natural products, and the owner runs free courses and lectures on various health subjects.

Springfield Pharmacy
124 Sheen Road
Richmond
Surrey KT5 9DZ
Tel: 020 8940 2304
Importers of sublingual and progesterone capsules and creams.

Well Woman's Information Service
BCM WWIN
LONDON WC1N 3XX
Tel: 07000 835994
email: info@wwin.cc

Natural Progesterone Information Packs are available by sending a first class stamp to the Well Woman's International Network, a free-to-join organisation. They have a fax consultation service for members directly with Dr Lee, distribute his monthly newsletter and organise his UK and Irish Seminars.

Simply Nature
Old Factory Buildings
Battenhurst Road
Stonegate TN5 7DU
Tel: 01580 201687

Organic and herbal skincare ranges, plus natural health and beauty products for the family.

NUTRITIONISTS AND THERAPISTS

Institute for Optimum Nutrition
Blades Court
Deodar Road
London SW15 2NU
Tel: 020 8877 9993

Educational trust running in-house and home-study courses. Has register of qualified nutrition consultants across the UK.

NS3UK
Centre for Nutrition Education
51 Trevelyan
Bracknell
Berkshire
RG12 8YD
Tel/Fax: 01344 360033
email enquiries@ns3.co.uk or visit www.ns3.co.uk

Directed by Kate Neil, a nutritionist specialising in hormonal health, and the author and editor of a professional
nutrition journal. NS3 provides consultations, professional
training courses and public workshops.

Penny Davenport
Nutritional Therapist
Battle
East Sussex
Tel: 01424 774103

Charlotte Bridge
Natural help for infertility
Tel: 01306 882 850

Hair tomorrow
Hair loss advice using natural methods including progesterone
Tel: 01628 776 5587

SUPPORT ORGANIZATIONS

CHILD
43 St Leonard's Road
Bexhill
East Sussex TN0 1JA
Tel: 01424 732361

National self-support group for those suffering from infertility.

Miscarriage Association
Clayton Hospital
Wakefield
West Yorkshire WF1 3JS
Tel: 01924 200799

Support and information on all aspects of pregnancy loss.

Breast Cancer Campaign
111 High Holborn
London WC1V 6JS
Tel: 020 7404 3955

Promotes and supports education and research into breast cancer.

Lavender Trust
Tel: 020 7384 2984

Breast cancer help for younger women.

PMS Support Services
Tel: 01279 427885

Leaflets, support and advice

Endometriosis Association
Suite 50, 1–7 Artillery Row
London SW1P 1RL
Helpline: 020 7222 2776

British Homoeopathic Association
27a Devonshire St
London WC1N 1RJ

National Institute of Medical Herbalists
34 Cambridge Road
London SW11

British Acupuncture Association and Register
34 Alderney Street
London SW1V 4EU
Tel: 020 7834 1012

RECOMMENDED READING

Dr John Lee, *What Your Doctor May Not Tell You About Menopause* (Warner Books)
Dr John Lee, *Multiple Roles of a Remarkable Hormone* (Jon Carpenter)
Kate Neil and Patrick Holford, *Balancing Hormones Naturally* (Piatkus)
Leslie Kenton, *Passage to Power* (Vermilion)
Kitty Campion, *Menopause Naturally* (Newleaf)
Christina Northrup, *Wisdom of the Menopause* (Piatkus)
Leslie Kenton, *Healing Herbs* (Ebury Press)

If you cannot find these titles in your local bookshop, all are available by mail order from Woman to Woman (see address above).

Index